1.95

KU-825-730

ANATOMY AND PHYSIOLOGY APPLIED TO NURSING

E07173

ANATOMY AND PHYSIOLOGY APPLIED TO NURSING

JANET T.E. RIDDLE RGN RFN ONC RNT(Edin)

Formerly Member of the Joint Examination Board,
British Orthopaedic Association and Central Council
for the Disabled. Formerly Senior Tutor, Western
District College of Nursing and Midwifery, Glasgow

Illustrated by Kathleen B. Nicoll RGN SCM ONC RCI(Edin) RNT DipAdEd

Formerly Senior Tutor, Western District College of
Nursing and Midwifery, Glasgow

SIXTH EDITION

Churchill Livingstone

EDINBURGH LONDON MELBOURNE AND NEW YORK 1985

CHURCHILL LIVINGSTONE
Medical Division of Longman Group UK Limited

Distributed in the United States of America by Churchill
Livingstone Inc., 1560 Broadway, New York, N.Y. 10036,
and by associated companies, branches and
representatives throughout the world.

First edition 1961
Second edition 1966
Third edition 1969
Fourth edition 1974
Fifth edition 1977
Sixth edition 1985
  Reprinted 1989

ISBN   0-443-03030-8

British Library Cataloguing in Publication Data
Riddle, Janet T.E.
   Anatomy and physiology applied to nursing.
   —6th ed.
   1. Human physiology
   I. Title
   612'.0024613   RT69

Library of Congress Cataloging in Publication Data
Riddle, Janet T.E.
   Anatomy and physiology applied to nursing.
   Rev. ed. of: Elementary textbook of anatomy and
physiology applied to nursing. 5th ed. 1977.
   Includes index.
   1. Anatomy, Human. 2. Human physiology.
3. Nursing. I. Riddle, Janet T.E. Elementary textbook of
anatomy and physiology applied to nursing. II. Title.
[DNLM: 1. Anatomy—nurses' instruction.
2. Physiology—nurses' instruction. QS 4 R543e]
RT69.R5   1985   611   84–21413

Produced by Longman Group (FE) Limited
Printed in Hong Hong

Preface to the Sixth Edition

In the twenty four years which have elapsed since this book was first published, medicine and nursing have evolved quite dramatically. The nurse of today must acquire a competent working knowledge of the structure and functions of the human body at an early stage in training. This elementary knowledge should enable the first year student to take an intelligent interest in the patient's condition and in the planning of total patient care.

The extensive revision of the text and its accompanying illustrations has been undertaken to meet the needs of the student during the first 18 months of training. The terminology has been revised to conform with international agreements, and study or revision questions have been included at the end of each chapter. These questions should reinforce learning and offer some practice for examination.

I wish to thank Miss Kathleen Nicoll for the work she has undertaken in improving and adding to the illustrations, Mrs Mary Emmerson Law of Churchhill Livingstone for her support and interest and Mrs M. Dickson for typing the script.

Glasgow, 1985   J.T.E.R.

Preface to the First Edition

This book is based on the lectures given to the nurses at Killearn Hospital during the first year of their training. During this year an attempt is made to give the student a simple overall picture of the human body and to make her apply her knowledge to the art of nursing which she is learning on the wards and in the classroom. The nurse, training for State Enrolment, requires no more than an elementary knowledge of anatomy and physiology. If these subjects are taught without practical application, they become the tedious and dreaded stumbling blocks to the passing of examinations. Applied to nursing, however, anatomy and physiology become interesting and alive and much that was bewildering becomes obvious.

The chapter on posture has been placed at the end of the book for ease of reference although its place is more rightly following Chapter 3. This is a subject which cannot be disposed of in one lecture, but must be taught over and over again particularly at the bedside.

I wish to express my grateful thanks to all who have helped in the preparation of this book; particularly Miss K. B. Nicoll who not only prepared the illustrations but typed the manuscript and assisted in the preparation of the material; Mr Athol Parkes for reading the manuscript; Professor Roland Barnes and Miss E. Macinnes for their helpful criticisms; Mr Charles Macmillan, Mr. James Parker and the staff of E. & S. Livingstone Ltd for the encouragement, advice and guidance which they have given so willingly. Many other friends as well as members of my family have contributed their help and encouragement and I am greatly indebted to them all.

Killearn, 1961   J.T.E.R.

Contents

Instructions for students

At the end of each chapter there are a variety of objective tests. These questions have been included so that you can assess your knowledge before going on to study the next system. The answers can be found on pages 187–191.

There are four different types of objective tests:

1. *Diagrams with numbered parts*. Beside each diagram is a list of lettered parts. Use this list to identify the numbered structures.

2 *Multiple choice questions*. Read the questions and from the four possible answers select the one which you think is correct.

3. *True/false questions*. These consist of a number of statements, some of which are true and some are false. Mark them 'T' for true and 'F' for false before checking with the answer list.

4. *Matching items questions*. These consist of two lists. On the left is a list of lettered items and on the right is a list of numbered items. Study the two lists and for each numbered item select the appropriate item from the lettered list.

1

Cells, tissues, organs and systems

Biology is the science which deals with all living things. *Anatomy* is the branch of biology which describes the structure of the body and the relationship of one part to another. *Physiology* is the study of how each part functions.

The human body is like a very complex and delicate machine, each minute part of which is constructed in such a way that it not only carries out its own functions but works as a whole with all the other parts. The nurse must learn to care for this machine and be able to detect when something goes wrong.

The purpose of this book is to help the nurse care for her patient. It is not possible, however, to nurse a patient adequately with only scientific knowledge. Nursing involves human understanding, providing for the emotional and spiritual needs of each patient and being able to work as a part of a team with other members of the caring professions.

THE CELLS

All living things are made of cells. The *amoeba* is one of the simplest of living organisms; it exists in water and consists of only one cell. We know that this shapeless creature is alive because, with the aid of a microscope, it can be seen to move, reproduce, grow and repair itself. It requires oxygen and food and can be seen to absorb this food and put out waste products. The amoeba can also react to its environment, moving away from its enemies and towards its food. Man also possesses all these characteristics but his body is a complex multicellular organism which takes nine months to grow into the form we recognise as human. He requires organs such as lungs, kidneys and bowels to perform what the amoeba does with one cell.

The human body is developed from the female egg cell or *ovum.* When the ovum is penetrated by the male germ cell (the *spermatozoon*) fusion takes place and one completely new cell called a *zygote* is formed. The zygote embeds itself in the wall of the womb and begins to multiply. The individual parts of the body result from the growth, development and multiplication of this cell during the nine months of pregnancy. As the cells multiply specialisation takes place, resulting in collections of cells with specific functions. These groupings of similar cells are called *tissues.*

All cells consist of a complex chemical compound called *protoplasm.* This gelatinous substance is composed largely of water with protein, sugar, fats and mineral salts in solution. It is contained within a fine semi-permeable membrane called the cell wall, through which the cell gets its nourishment and expels its waste.

Cells require a fluid environment. This fluid, which surrounds all the cells, is called *tissue fluid.* There is a constant interchange between the water in the cell (intracellular) and the water in the tissues (extracellular). Because the cell wall is semi-permeable, substances in solution pass in and out of the cell as required.

The cell must receive the correct amount of water, oxygen and nutrients, no less and no more than is necessary to carry out the complex chemical reactions which take place in the protoplasm. Imagine that each cell is a small factory. If it is to work efficiently there must be a continuous delivery of raw materials, sale of the manufactured product and removal of the accumulated waste. If a strike stops any of these three processes the factory will grind to a halt. Similarly, in man, if he is deprived of food and water for a long enough period he will become weak and drowsy and

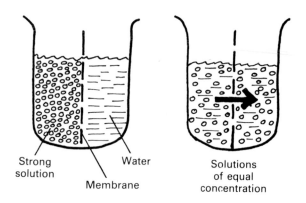

Fig. 1.1 Diffusion

unconsciousness may result. His cells have got clogged up with waste, the flow of nutrients is disrupted and the work of the cells comes to a halt.

The volume and composition of intracellular and extracellular fluids must be kept constant. The main processes involved are called diffusion, osmosis and filtration.

Diffusion occurs when substances in solution have a molecule which is small enough to pass through the tiny pores in the cell membrane. Diffused substances pass from the stronger to the weaker solution.

Osmosis is the process which draws water through a semi-permeable membrane from the weaker to the stronger solution. It is of the utmost importance in all living activities.

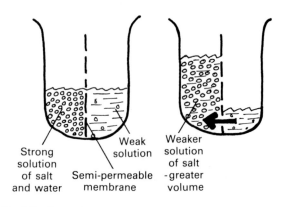

Fig. 1.2 Osmosis

Filtration occurs when the pressures on either side of the cell wall are different. The greater pressure forces fluid through the membrane to the other side.

On microscopic examination the cells are seen to contain a variety of different shaped structures. Some of these are *granules* which are nutrient substances, others are clear spaces called *vacuoles* which may contain waste substances or digestive enzymes. In the centre is a dense structure called the *nucleus* which has a round body near it called the *centrosome*. This centrosome is concerned with cell division.

Inside the nucleus there are threadlike structures which carry *genes*. Genes, which are composed of deoxyribonucleic acid commonly known as DNA, transmit characteristics from one generation to the next. The threadlike structures which contain the genes are called *chromosomes* and each human cell has 46 chromosomes arranged in 23 pairs, the two parts of each pair being identical. When a cell divides, the chromosomes split in two lengthwise. The two daughter cells which result contain the same number of chromosomes and therefore the same genes as the parent cell.

Cell division is most active in fetal life and during the growing period. Although some cells eventually lose this ability to divide some continue to reproduce throughout life. This is particularly important when the tissues are subjected to wear and tear or when cells are destroyed as a result of injury. In some way, the rate of growth and reproduction is controlled. If anything goes wrong with this mechanism and cell production goes out of control abnormal growths or tumours are formed.

The sex cells differ in their method of division. In this case the chromosomes do not split but one of each pair of chromosomes goes to the daughter cells. These cells are called *gametes* and they contain only 23 chromosomes, half the normal number. When the ovum and the sperm fuse to form the new life the resulting *zygote* contains 46 chromosomes, 23 from each parent, and the child inherits the characteristics of both parents. These inherited characteristics include hair colour, but obviously the offspring of a red-headed mother and a black-haired father does not inherit red and black hair. This is because some genes are recessive and some are dominant. If the baby has red hair his mother's gene for hair colour has been dominant and his father's recessive. This also accounts for the differences and similarities in the charac-

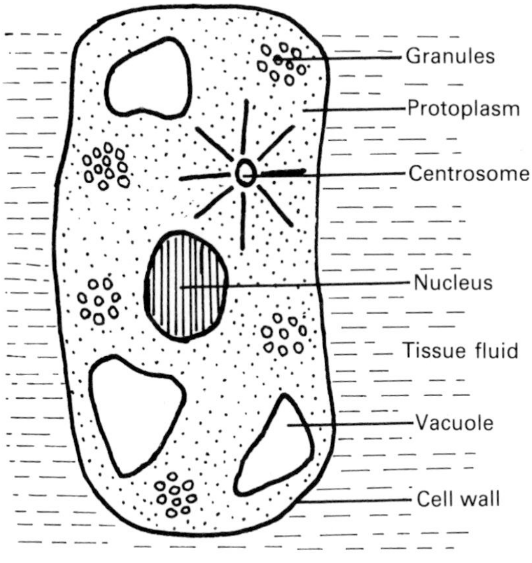

Fig. 1.3 A Cell

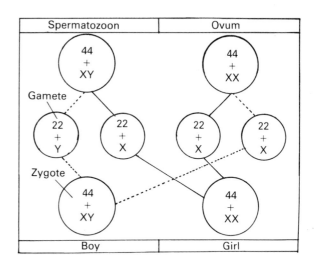

Fig. 1.4

teristics of the children of one family. The fact that certain characteristics may reappear having missed one or more generations is due to the recessive genes having become dominant.

The sex of the child depends on the sex chromosomes. The female cell nucleus contains a matching pair called the XX sex chromosomes. The male cell nucleus contains a pair which are not identical called the XY sex chromosomes. As you can see from Figure 1.4, if the ovum is fertilised by a sperm containing the X chromosome the baby will be a girl but if it contains the Y chromosome it will be a boy.

THE TISSUES

If the cells are the building bricks of the body, the tissues must be the walls. This is not a very good analogy because it suggests that all tissues are firm and hard whereas the only really hard tissues are bone and teeth. We have already seen that cells are soft and gelatinous, consisting mainly of water, and that they are living and constantly changing. Examining a bone from the skeleton will not help you to visualise the tissues, but purchase a piece of meat from the butcher and separate the different materials with a pair of forceps. You will see muscle and fat tissues and tissues which look as if they were woven from threads. If you have a microscope available you will see the cells.

Cells are of different shapes and sizes: some are globular, some like columns or cubes, and others flat like paving stones. They are joined together to form walls, coverings, tubes, sheets and packing material. The resulting tissues form different parts of the body and behave differently.

There are four main classifications of cells—*epithelial, connective, muscle* and *nervous*—therefore there are four types of tissue, each with subdivisions.

The diagrams which follow will give you some idea of how these tissues look under the microscope.

Epithelial tissues

Epithelial tissues form the covering of the body and the lining of various organs. The cells are cemented closely together and there are several types. Simple epithelium consists of one layer of cells. Compound epithelium is several layers thick.

Squamous epithelium

This consists of a single layer of flat cells. It provides a smooth lining for the heart and blood vessels and is also present in the lungs.

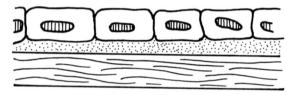

Fig. 1.5 Squamous epithelium

Cuboid epithelium

This consists of cube-shaped cells which secrete and absorb substances. It forms part of the kidney.

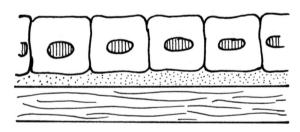

Fig. 1.6 Cuboid epithelium

Columnar epithelium

This is a single layer of column-shaped cells which secrete mucus. This tissue is commonly called *mucous membrane* and is found lining the food passages. Mucus is a viscid lubricat-

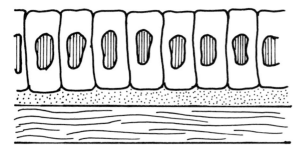

Fig. 1.7 Columnar epithelium

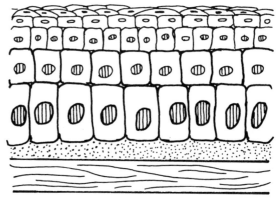

Fig. 1.9 Stratified epithelium

ing fluid which helps to move the food along. Some of the cells of this tissue absorb food substances.

Ciliated columnar epithelium

This lines the respiratory passages. It has fine hair-like processes called cilia on the free surface of the cells. These cilia sweep the mucus containing dust particles away from the lungs and into the throat.

and parts of the mouth. It will stand up to considerable wear and tear as the deep cells replace the superficial cells by division.

Transitional epithelium

This occurs in the bladder and consists of three layers of pear-shaped cells.

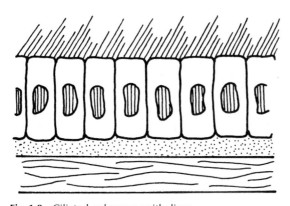

Fig. 1.8 Ciliated columnar epithelium

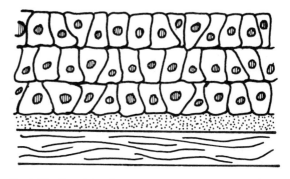

Fig. 1.10 Transitional epithelium

Stratified epithelium

This consists of several layers of cells which vary in shape. The deepest layers are column-shaped and the surface layers are flattened. This tissue forms the outer layers of the skin

Glands

These are structures consisting of secreting epithelial cells, some of which have ducts through which they pour their secretion while others are ductless. The ductless glands put their secretions, called hormones, straight into the blood stream.

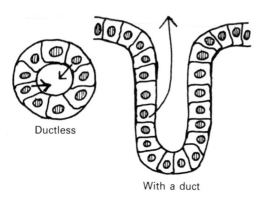

Ductless

With a duct

Fig. 1.11 Glands

Connective tissues

The cells of the connective tissues produce a secretion which forms a ground substance or matrix. This matrix may be soft, semi-solid or rigid and may contain fibres which are thread-like structures. There is a considerable amount of matrix which means that the cells are quite widely spaced. Connective tissues are supporting tissues, binding, covering and protecting other tissues. The student will find it advantageous to have a specimen of a joint from the butcher before starting to study these tissues.

Loose connective tissue—areolar tissue

This tissue is widely distributed throughout the body. It is found under the skin and supporting and covering the muscles, blood vessels and nerves. It consists of a soft matrix containing a network of fibres.

Adipose tissue

This is similar to loose connective tissue but contains an abundance of fat cells. It is found under the skin surrounding the kidneys, behind the eyes and in the marrow of bones.

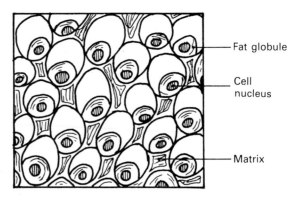

Fat globule

Cell nucleus

Matrix

Fig. 1.13 Adipose tissue

White fibrous tissue

This is a tough tissue with very little matrix and few cells but many bundles of white fibres. It forms the ligaments which tie bones together and the tendons which tie muscle to bone. It also forms protective coverings for many organs.

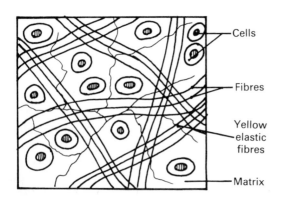

Cells

Fibres

Yellow elastic fibres

Matrix

Fig. 1.12 Loose connective tissue

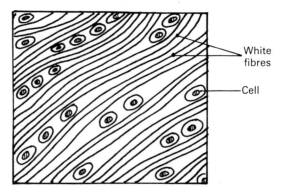

White fibres

Cell

Fig. 1.14 White fibrous tissue

Yellow elastic fibrous tissue

This is similar to white fibrous tissue but the fibres are more elastic and are yellow in colour. It is found in the formation of the walls of arteries and in the lungs. These are organs which must be able to stretch and recoil.

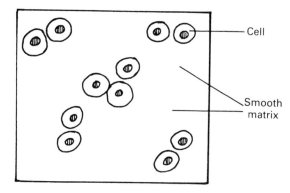

Fig. 1.16 Hyaline cartilage

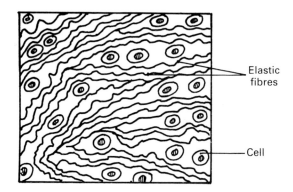

Fig. 1.15 Yellow elastic fibrous tissue

Lymphoid tissue

This is a specialised tissue found in the lymphatic system.

Blood

This is a connective tissue with a fluid matrix and will be described in Chapter 4.

Cartilage and bone

These are the connective tissues of the skeleton. In early fetal life the greater part of the skeleton is cartilage, but this is gradually replaced by bone until in adult life the only remaining cartilage is found forming joints, in the chest wall, in the respiratory system and in the nose and ears. Cartilage has a firm elastic matrix and there are three types.

Hyaline cartilage

Hyaline cartilage which has a smooth matrix is bluish white in appearance and is found cov-

ering the ends of bone involved in joint formation.

White fibro-cartilage and yellow elastic fibro-cartilage

These differ from hyaline cartilage in that the matrix contains dense bundles of white or yellow elastic fibres. White fibro-cartilage forms the discs of the spine and yellow elastic fibrocartilage forms the ears and the walls of the respiratory passages.

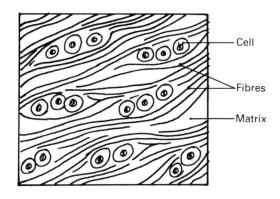

Fig. 1.17 White fibrocartilage

Bone

This has a hard matrix and will be described in Chapter 2.

Muscle tissue

There are three types of muscle tissue:
  voluntary, skeletal or striated
  involuntary, visceral or plain
  cardiac

Voluntary muscle tissue

This tissue forms the muscles which are responsible for the movement of the skeleton. It is under the control of the will, hence the name voluntary. The cells are elongated and striated or striped with light and dark bands. They may contain many nuclei.

Involuntary muscle tissue

This tissue has elongated cells but no stripes. It is found forming the walls of internal organs (viscera) which are not under direct control of the will.

Cardiac muscle tissue

This is the muscle tissue of the heart and is not found anywhere else in the body. It is not under control of the will. The cells are elongated, striated and branched and contain only one nucleus.

Nervous tissue

This is the tissue which forms the brain, the spinal cord and the nerves. It is a soft tissue, grey and white in colour and will be described in more detail in Chapter 9.

SYSTEMS AND ORGANS

The body is composed of nine different systems. A system is a collection of organs and an organ is a collection of tissues. Take the heart as an example. This is an organ of the circulatory system. It is made of cardiac muscle tissue because its function is a pumping movement. It is lined with squamous epithelium to give the blood a smooth surface over which to flow and is covered by tough fibrous tissue which protects it.

Each system carries out one or more of the vital functions of the body but none of the systems can work independently.

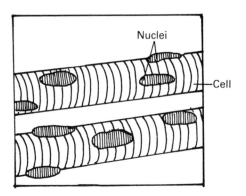

Fig. 1.18 Voluntary muscle tissue

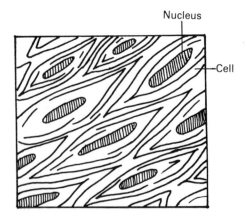

Fig. 1.19 Involuntary muscle tissue

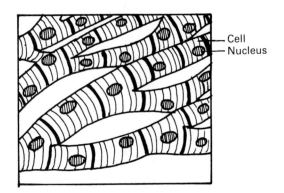

Fig. 1.20 Cardiac muscle tissue

The systems

The skeletal system

The *bones* of the skeletal system form a framework which gives the body its shape. In some cases the bones act as a protective covering for delicate organs.

The muscular system

The *muscles* are attached to the skeleton and produce movement.

The circulatory system

The organs of the circulatory system are the *heart* and *blood vessels* which carry nourishment to all the cells of the body and the *spleen* and *lymphatic* vessels which help to combat infection.

The respiratory system

The *lungs* and *air passages* make up the respiratory system. Its function is to take in air rich in oxygen and to expel air containing carbon dioxide.

The digestive system

This consists of the *alimentary canal*, the *liver*, the *pancreas* and the *salivary glands*. The alimentary canal is made up of the *mouth, pharynx, oesophagus, stomach* and *bowel*. The function is ingestion, digestion and absorption of food.

The urinary or excretory system

This system consists of the *kidneys* which secrete waste, the *ureters* which carry it to the *bladder* to be stored and the *urethra* through which it is excreted. The word excretion means the elimination of waste material from the body. This is also a function of the large intestine and lungs and one of the many functions of the skin.

The nervous system

The *brain, spinal cord* and *nerves* make up the nervous system which is responsible for co-ordinating the work of other systems and for interaction with the external environment. Closely associated with the nervous system are the *skin, ears, eyes* and *nose*. These are the organs which receive sensations from the environment and relay them to the brain.

The endocrine system

This consists of various *glands* which produce *hormones*. Hormones are chemical substances which regulate the body's activities.

The reproductive systems

These systems are concerned with the continuity of the human race and consist of the *uterus, ovaries* and *vagina* in the female and the *testes* and *penis* in the male.

THE ANATOMICAL PARTS OF THE BODY

The body can be divided into four parts—the head, the neck, the trunk and the limbs.

The head

The bony framework of the head is the skull. The skull contains several cavities, the largest of which is the *cranium* containing the brain. The other cavities are the nose (nasal), the mouth (oral) and the orbits (orbital) which contain the eyes.

The neck

The neck joins the head to the trunk and consists of part of the spinal column and the food and the air passages passing down into the trunk.

The trunk

The trunk is divided into three cavities:
   the thorax or thoracic cavity
   the abdomen or abdominal cavity
   the pelvis or pelvic cavity

The thorax

The uppermost cavity is the thorax or chest. The boundaries of this cavity are the spinal column, the ribs, the breast bone and the diaphragm. The *diaphragm* is a thin sheet of mus-

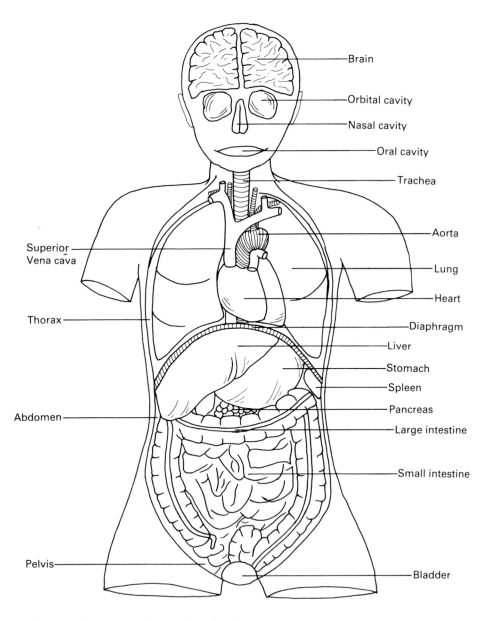

Fig. 1.21 Head, neck and trunk showing organs and cavities

cle tissue which forms the floor of the thorax and separates it from the abdomen. This cavity contains the lungs, the heart, large blood vessels and the oesophagus.

The abdomen

The abdomen is the largest of the cavities. At the back is the spine and in front a large powerful group of muscles which not only hold the organs in place but help to support the body in the upright position. The abdominal organs are the stomach, the bowel (intestines), the liver, the pancreas, the spleen and the kidneys. This cavity is divided into nine regions so that the positions of these organs can be identified.

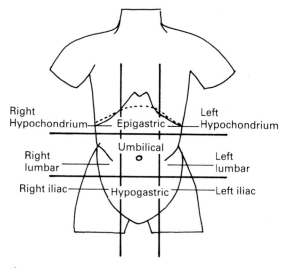

Fig. 1.22 Regions of the abdomen

The pelvis

The pelvis is a funnel-shaped cavity with bony walls. It contains the reproductive organs, the ureters and urinary bladder, and the lower part of the bowel.

The limbs

The upper and lower limbs are appendages attached to the trunk and give the individual independence. They consist of bone covered by the muscles which produce movement. Blood vessels and nerves run through these structures.

Cells, tissues, organs and systems questions

Diagrams—Questions 1–20

1–5 A cell

  A. Cell wall
  B. Nucleus
  C. Granule
  D. Centrosome
  E. Protoplasm

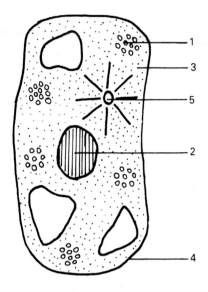

```
1
2
3
4
5
```

6–14. Head, neck and trunk

  A. Diaphragm
  B. Bladder
  C. Heart
  D. Intestine
  E. Liver
  F. Lungs
  G. Pancreas
  H. Stomach
  I. Thorax

```
6
7
8
9
10
11
12
13
14
```

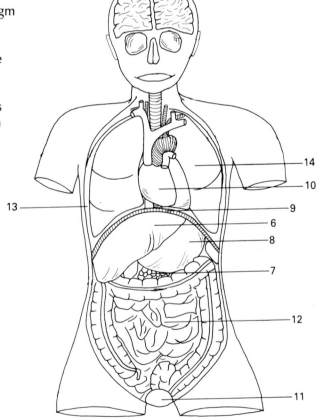

15–20 **Regions of the abdomen**

    A. Hypogastric region

    B. Epigastric region

    C. Left hypochondriac region

    D. Left iliac region

    E. Left lumbar region

    F. Umbilical region

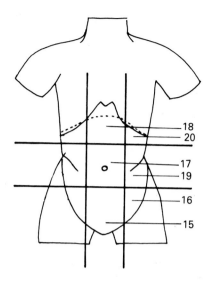

15
16
17
18
19
20

Questions 21–35 are of the multiple choice type

21. Which one of the following parts of a cell contains the genes?
    A. Centrosome
    B. Chromosome
    C. Granule
    D. Vacuole.

21

22. Zygote is the name given to :
    A. the female egg cell
    B. the fertilised ovum
    C. the male sex cell
    D. all sex cells.

22

23. Osmosis occurs when :
    A. increased pressure forces a solution through a membrane
    B. a concentrated solution draws fluid from a weak solution
    C. solids pass across a semi-permeable membrane
    D. water passes across a permeable membrane.

23

24. The number of chromosomes in each ordinary human cell is:
    A. 22
    B. 23
    C. 44
    D. 46.

24

25. The number of chromosomes in a gamete is:
    A. 22
    B. 23
    C. 44
    D. 46.

25

26. Tissues :
    A. are all soft in consistency
    B. consist of a number of different cells
    C. consist of a number of similar cells
    D. have only one function.

26

27. Epithelium is the tissue which forms :
    A. coverings for organs
    B. linings for organs
    C. walls of organs
    D. tendons and ligaments.

27

28. **Which one of the following epithelial tissues forms the outer part of the skin?**
    A. Ciliated
    B. Cuboid
    C. Stratified
    D. Transitional.

29. **Which one of the following is not a connective tissue?**
    A. Blood
    B. Bone
    C. Cartilage
    D. Muscle.

30. **Tendons :**
    A. are made of areolar tissue
    B. are made of white fibro-cartilage
    C. join muscle to bone
    D. join bone to bone.

31. **Hyaline cartilage :**
    A. has a soft matrix
    B. contains calcium
    C. forms part of the structure of a bone
    D. forms ligaments.

32. **Voluntary muscle tissue cells are :**
    A. branched
    B. plain
    C. striped
    D. striped and branched.

33. **Which one of the following organs is part of the circulatory system?**
    A. Pancreas
    B. Spleen
    C. Pharynx
    D. Lungs.

34. **Which one of the following organs does not excrete waste?**
    A. Pancreas
    B. Kidneys
    C. Lungs
    D. Skin.

35. **A hormone is :**
    A. part of a cell
    B. a chemical product of a gland
    C. part of the nervous system
    D. a gland with a duct.

2

The skeletal system

The skeleton is the framework which gives the body its shape. In the human body it consists of an axis—the bones of the head and trunk, and four appendages—the arms and legs. Covering the bones are muscles and skin. Muscle is a remarkably resilient tissue but skin and fibrous tissue are more easily affected by adverse circumstances. If the bones are well covered by muscle they do not present a nursing problem. However, where bony prominences lie just under the skin they become important as pressure points when the patient is unable to move himself freely. Friction and pressure over these bony parts limits the blood supply to the skin causing death of tissue. Some knowledge of the structure of the skeleton is, therefore, necessary so that the nurse knows which areas of skin are vulnerable.

The bones are made up of several different tissues and have different shapes. On examining the skeleton one would think that there were many differently shaped bones, but each bone belongs to one of only four categories: long, short, flat and irregular.

Long bones

The long bones provide the framework of the limbs, and because of their shape and method of attachment to each other they allow movement. Each long bone has a tubular shaft with a central cavity (called the medullary canal) and two rounded extremities. The bones of

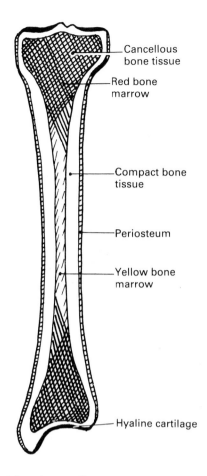

Fig. 2.1   A long bone—tibia

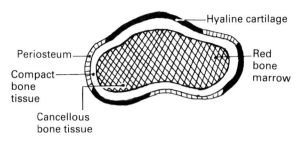

Fig. 2.2   A short bone—talus

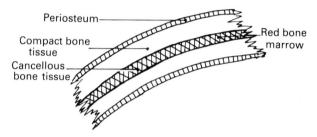

Fig. 2.3   A flat bone—skull

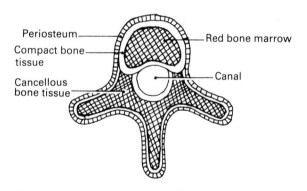

Fig. 2.4   An irregular bone—vertebra

the fingers and toes are also classified as long bones since, although they are very small, they have the same shape.

Short bones

The short bones have no uniform shape. They are collected together in groups at the wrists and the ankles, forming units strong enough to support the weight of the body.

Flat bones

The bones of the skull, thorax and pelvis are flat bones. They form the walls of the major body cavities and protect their contents.

Irregular bones

The vertebrae and bones of the face are irregular in form. They cannot be classified with any of the other groups.

THE STRUCTURE OF BONES

The tissues which form the bones are:
    bone tissue (compact and cancellous)
    fibrous tissue
    hyaline cartilage
    adipose tissue

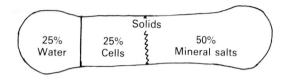

Fig. 2.5 Composition of bone

These are all connective tissues. Studying a dried classroom bone specimen gives quite the wrong impression and makes it difficult to appreciate that a bone is a living, constantly changing, organism consisting of 25% water and 75% solids. Living bone cells and other organic material account for 1/3rd of the solids. The rest is made up of mineral salts, mainly *calcium* and *phosphorus*, which therefore account for 50% of the total bone composition.

Examination of the dried specimen shows roughened areas where muscles, tendons and ligaments were attached. We can also see smooth areas where joints were formed and grooves for the passage of blood vessels and nerves.

Bone tissue

There are two types of bone tissue, an inner spongy or *cancellous* bone and a hard outer *compact* bone.

The cancellous tissue looks like a sponge and is full of little spaces surrounded by thin plates of bone. It is present in the extremities of the long bones, in the centre of short bones and sandwiched between the compact plates of the flat bones.

The compact bone tissue forms a shell which varies in thickness and gives the bone its strength. When it is examined by the naked eye it appears to be solid, but under the microscope it is seen to consist of little plates of bone as in cancellous bone tissue. However, in compact bone tissue the plates are closer together and are arranged in a concentric manner. Between these plates, called lamellae, is fluid containing the bone cells. These cells are called *osteophytes*.

Fibrous tissue

A sheet of fibrous tissue adheres to all the surfaces of each bone except for the smooth areas where joints are formed. It provides a protective covering which helps in the nourishment and growth of the bone. It is called the *periosteum.*

Through the periosteum run small blood vessels carrying food, calcium and oxygen to the bone cells. If you examine the bone carefully you will see small 'scratches' on the shaft. These are, in fact, openings through which the blood vessels enter the bone.

Hyaline cartilage

Hyaline cartilage is a bluish white translucent tissue which is smooth like glass. It is found at the extremities of long bones and wherever there is a movable joint. This tissue is sometimes referred to as *articular cartilage* and it allows the bones to glide freely on each other.

Adipose tissue—red and yellow bone marrow

Red bone marrow is the fatty tissue found in the spaces in cancellous bone tissue. This tissue has a very important function to play as it is here that the blood cells are developed and matured before they are released into the blood stream.

Infants up to the age of 5 years have red bone marrow in the medullary canals of their long bones. This is gradually replaced by yellow marrow which contains more fat cells and fewer blood cells.

THE GROWTH AND DEVELOPMENT OF BONE

The growth and development of bone is influenced by the action of hormones from certain ductless (endocrine) glands and by the amount of *calcium phosphate* and *vitamin D* in the diet. Milk, cheese, eggs and green vegetables contain calcium which makes the bone hard. Vitamin D, which is found in animal fats and cod liver oil, regulates the use the body makes of calcium. This vitamin is manufactured in the skin when it is exposed to the ultra violet rays of the sun.

The fetal skeleton is made of tough flexible cartilage. This is gradually hardened by the laying down of calcium which, in the presence of vitamin D, has been absorbed from the food and carried in the blood stream to the skeleton. This process is called *ossification* and is not completed in all bones until the individual reaches the early twenties when all growth finally stops. The diet must contain sufficient calcium and vitamin D for this process and this is particularly important in the case of pregnant women and growing children.

Figure 2.6 shows the development of a long bone from a small rod of cartilage in early fetal life to a fully developed bone. Bone building cells called osteoblasts remove calcium from the blood stream and lay it down as small plates in the cartilage. The process starts in the middle of the shaft of a long bone at the *primary centre* of *ossification*. From this centre calcium is laid down in both directions forming the shaft or *diaphysis*. As ossification takes place the diaphysis gets longer. Sometime after birth, *secondary centres* develop at the ends of the bone. The ossified extremities are called the *epiphyses*. Between the epiphysis and the diaphysis is a plate of cartilage, called the *epiphyseal cartilage*, which is the growing area of the bone. This cartilage is present until growth stops and can be seen on an X-ray plate as a space between the shaft and the extremity.

Malabsorption of calcium and vitamin D at any age or their absence in the diet will result in softening of the bones. In children the deficiency results in rickets. The bones become pliable and will bend as they bear the increasing weight of the child. Knock knees or bowed legs result, but fortunately this condition is now uncommon in this country.

Broken bones are not common in young children and when they do occur the bone

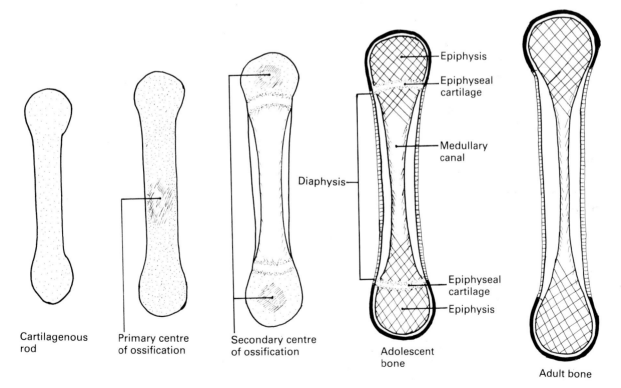

Cartilagenous rod

Primary centre of ossification

Secondary centre of ossification

Diaphysis

Epiphysis

Epiphyseal cartilage

Medullary canal

Epiphyseal cartilage

Epiphysis

Adolescent bone

Adult bone

Fig. 2.6 Development of a long bone

snaps on one side and then tears lengthwise, like breaking young twigs in the spring. This is called a green-stick fracture. As one grows older the bones become progressively harder, and in old age they may become quite brittle so that a trivial injury can produce a fracture. A bone is said to be fractured when it is broken into two or more pieces.

THE BONES OF THE SKELETON

The skeleton is made up of a number of parts. The bones of the head and trunk form the central support or axial skeleton. The upper limbs, which are attached to the trunk by the shoulder girdle, and the lower limbs, which are at-

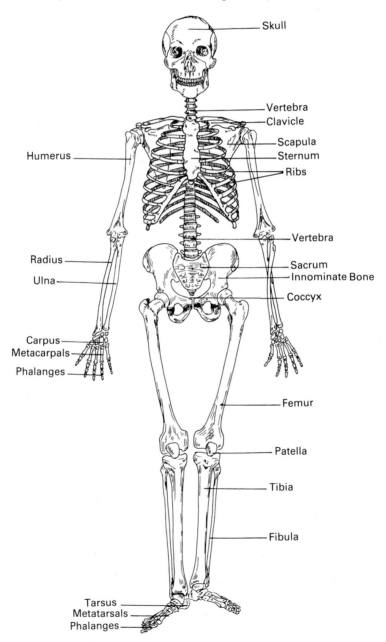

Skull

Vertebra
Clavicle
Scapula
Sternum
Ribs

Humerus

Vertebra

Sacrum
Innominate Bone
Coccyx

Radius
Ulna

Carpus
Metacarpals
Phalanges

Femur

Patella

Tibia

Fibula

Tarsus
Metatarsals
Phalanges

Fig. 2.7 The bones of the skeleton

tached to the pelvic girdle, form the appendicular skeleton.

Before going on to study the individual bones the following descriptive terms must be understood.

ANATOMICAL TERMS

1. The *anatomical position* is standing upright with the face looking forward, the legs straight with the feet together. The arms are held by the side with the palms of the hands facing the front.
2. The *midline* is an imaginary line drawn through the centre of the body from the crown of the head to the feet.
3. *Superior* means above.
4. *Inferior* means below.
5. *Anterior* means in front.
6. *Posterior* means behind.
7. *Lateral* means furthest from the midline.
8. *Medial* means nearest to the midline.
9. *Proximal* means the part of a limb nearest to its point of attachment to the body.
10. *Distal* means the part of a limb furthest away from its point of attachment.
11. *Supine* means lying on the back with the face up. It also means palm up.
12. *Prone* means lying face down or palm down.
13. An *articulation* means the joining of two or more bones.
14. A *foramen* is a hole through a bone.

THE SPINE OR VERTEBRAL COLUMN

The human animal is a vertebrate. This means that he has a back bone. This is not one long bone extending from the head to the tail but a series of small irregular bones. These bones are attached to each other in such a way that the spine can carry out its function as a central support for the body and at the same time remain mobile.

There are 33 vertebrae and, with a few exceptions, they are similar in structure. Each one has a box shaped *body* which lies in front

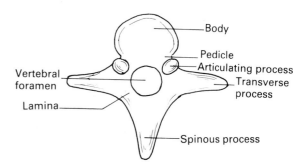

Fig. 2.8 A typical vertebra

and takes the weight. Projecting backwards from this is an arch of bone called the neural or *vertebral arch*. This arch encloses an opening, called the vertebral foramen, which is part of the canal through which the spinal cord passes. The spinal cord carries the nerves from the brain to all parts of the body.

The arch is joined to the body by the *pedicles* and has three projecting *processes* to which are attached the muscles which move the vertebral column. Each vertebra can move on its neighbour because of the little joints between the *articulating processes* on the laminae. The *laminae* are the flat pieces of bone which form the back of the arch. The prominent *spinous processes* can be felt all the way down the spine. These form important pressure areas when the patient has to be nursed supine.

The regions and curves of the spine

If the spine is viewed from the side it will be seen that it is not straight but forms four curves. These curves are not all present at birth but gradually develop as the infant 'unfolds', lifts its head up to look around, sits up on its mother's knee, crawls, stands up and eventually takes its first steps. When the baby is born and for the first few weeks of life, the spine consists of one continuous curve so that he is curled up like a ball. As his brain develops, so does the desire to see what is going on. He looks upwards and a secondary curve appears in the neck. This is the *cervical curve*. By the time he has reached the stage of pulling himself up from all fours to the upright pos-

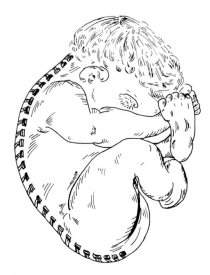

Fig. 2.9 The spinal curve at birth

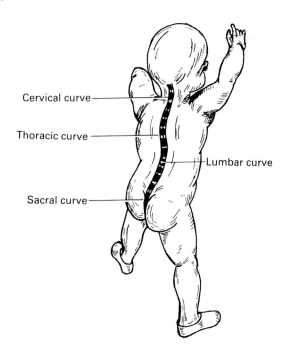

Fig. 2.11 The curves of the spine

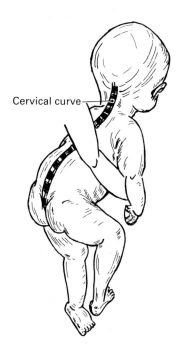

Fig. 2.10

ition and learns to balance, a further curve has developed in the small of his back. This is the *lumbar curve*.

The vertebrae are grouped into five regions. These regions relate to the curves and consist of:

the cervical vertebrae—the neck
the thoracic vertebrae—the back
the lumbar vertebrae—the loin
the sacral vertebrae—the pelvis
the coccygeal vertebrae—the tail

The bones forming each part of the spine are slightly different. They can be distinguished by their size and shape. The bones in the neck are small, but they become progressively larger until the pelvis is reached, then smaller again to form the tail.

The cervical vertebrae

There are seven cervical vertebrae. They are smaller than the rest and have three openings: the vertebral foramen and two smaller holes through which pass blood vessels going up to the brain.

The first two cervical vertebrae are called the *atlas* and the *axis*.

The *atlas* is a ring of bone with no body but a large foramen for the beginning of the spinal cord. It articulates with the skull and because of its shape allows the nodding movements of the head.

Anterior   Posterior

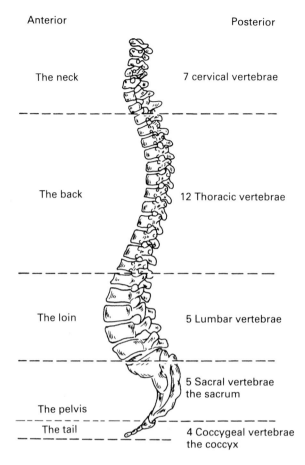

The neck   7 cervical vertebrae

The back   12 Thoracic vertebrae

The loin   5 Lumbar vertebrae

5 Sacral vertebrae the sacrum

The pelvis

The tail   4 Coccygeal vertebrae the coccyx

Fig. 2.12 The regions and curves of the spine

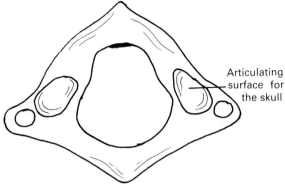

Articulating surface for the skull

Fig. 2.14 The atlas

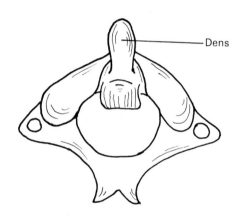

Dens

Fig. 2.15 The axis

The thoracic vertebrae

There are twelve thoracic vertebrae. They form the back of the thorax and have the ribs attached to them. They are slightly larger than the cervical vertebrae because they carry more weight. The spinous processes project downwards. They are very pointed and because of the backwards curve of the spine in this region can be easily felt under the skin.

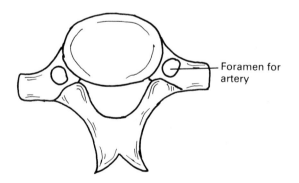

Foramen for artery

Fig. 2.13 A cervical vertebra

The *axis* has a tooth-like process called the *dens*, which projects upwards from its body. This is the pivot round which the atlas and the skull rotate allowing the shaking movements of the head.

The lumbar vertebrae

There are five lumbar vertebrae. They have the largest bodies and the smallest foramina. The spinous processes are thicker and less pointed but they are still easily identified in the lower part of the body.

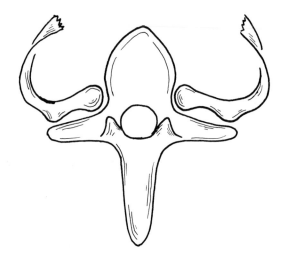

Fig. 2.16 Thoracic vertebra with ribs attached

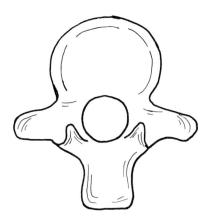

Fig. 2.17 A lumbar vertebra

The sacrum

There are five sacral vertebrae fused together to form a triangular-shaped bone called the sacrum. This bone is wedged between the innominate bones at the back of the pelvis. The foramina in this bone are for the passage of nerves (see Fig. 2.28).

There is very little muscle over the sacrum, and when sitting or lying in a chair or a bed this area is subjected to a considerable amount of pressure and friction. It is important to examine this area and to move the patient frequently to prevent the formation of bed sores.

The coccyx

The last four vertebrae form the coccyx. They are not properly formed and are fused together. The coccyx has no function in the human but is the tail in the lower animals (see Fig. 2.28).

Functions of the vertebral column

The functions of the vertebral column are *protection*, *support* and *movement*.

The last two functions seem to contradict each other because we know that the best type of support is something rigid. However, a series of ligaments, muscles and intervertebral discs allow the vertebral column to be both rigid and mobile.

Protection

The delicate spinal cord extends the whole length of the vertebral canal from the first cervical vertebra to the lumbar region, yet the spine can be bent and twisted without harming it.

Holding the vertebrae together and preventing them from slipping off each other are a series of ligaments. These act as ties and

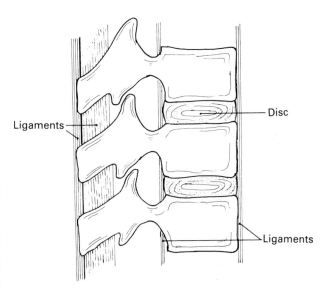

Fig. 2.18 Lateral view of spine showing discs and ligaments

allow the necessary range of safe movement and no more. In any injury to the neck or back these ligaments may be torn, allowing the vertebrae to move away from each other and thus disrupting the continuous canal and damaging the cord. Anyone rendering first aid to a patient with a history of having hurt his back must remember this and move the patient very carefully. Such patients should be kept flat and, if they must be moved, they should be rolled or lifted in one piece and never bent in the middle.

The spinal cord carries the nerves from the brain to all parts of the body so an injury to it may result in *tetraplegia* or *paraplegia*. In these conditions there is paralysis of all the muscles below the level of the injury to the spinal cord.

Support

The vertebral column acts as a support for the body. This is possible because of the shape of the bones and the presence of ligaments and muscles. There are groups of muscles attached to the spine for the whole of its length. These produce the movements which allow the spine to be fixed in whatever position is desired so that it may act as a rigid support.

Movement

The spine is very mobile, permitting a wide range of forward, backward, side-to-side and twisting movements. These movements are possible because there are small freely movable joints between the laminae of all the vertebrae. Discs of specialised tissue lie between the vertebral bodies, acting as cushions and shock absorbers. These *intervertebral discs* are rather like the sorbo rubber cushion or air ring between the patient and the mattress, allowing him just enough movement to vary the area of pressure from one point of his buttock to another. Discs, like cushions, sometimes get torn and the soft inner part leaks out. This protrusion causes pressure on the nerves as they leave the cord. The resulting pain is one symptom connected with the so-called 'slipped disc.'

THE SKULL

The skull is described in two parts: the cranium and the face.

The cranium

The cranium is the bony box which contains and protects the brain. It consists of eight, mainly flat bones joined together to form the walls of the cranial cavity.

The frontal bone

The frontal bone forms the forehead and the roof of the orbits. The orbits are the cone-shaped cavities which contain the eyes.

The parietal bones

There are two parietal bones forming the top or vault of the cranium.

(a)

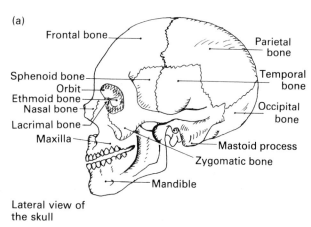

Lateral view of the skull

(b)

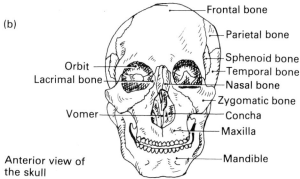

Anterior view of the skull

Fig. 2.19 The skull

The temporal bones

The temporal bones contain the internal parts of the ears. On the outside of the bone can be seen the opening into the *ear*. Behind this lies the prominent mastoid process to which some of the muscles moving the head are attached. This thick piece of bone contains air spaces which communicate with the ear. Below the ear is the articulating surface for the jaw.

The occipital bone

The occipital bone forms the back of the base of the cranium. It contains a large opening called the *foramen magnum*. This is where the spinal cord leaves the brain to pass down the vertebral or neural canal. On either side of this opening are two oval articulating surfaces where the skull forms a joint with the atlas. Nodding of the head is brought about by movement at this joint.

The sphenoid bone

The sphenoid bone is an irregular bone shaped like a bat. If forms part of the base or floor of the cranium. There are two openings in the sphenoid called the *optic foramina* through which the optic nerves pass from the eyes to the brain.

The ethmoid bone

The ethmoid bone is an irregular bone shaped like a box. It forms the bony framework of the *nose*. The top of the box is perforated for the passage of the nerve of smell (olfactory nerve).

The face

The skeleton of the face consists of thirteen irregular bones arranged in such a way that they form the orbits, part of the nose and the walls of the mouth or oral cavity.

The zygomatic (malar) bone

The zygomatic bones are the cheek bones. They help to form the orbits.

The maxilla

The maxilla is the upper jaw. It contains the upper teeth and forms part of the roof of the mouth.

The mandible

The mandible is the lower jaw. This bone contains the lower teeth and is attached to the temporal bone by two freely movable joints which can be felt in front of the ear when chewing.

The nasal bones

The nasal bones form the bridge of the nose.

The lacrimal bones

The lacrimal bones are very small bones situated in the inner corner of each orbit. They form a passage for the tear ducts.

The inferior concha (turbinates) and vomer

The inferior concha and vomer form part of the walls and the septum of the nose.

The palatine bones

The palatine bones form the roof of the mouth or palate.

The joints of the skull

The joints of the skull, with the exception of the joint between the mandible and the temporal bones, are immovable joints called *sutures*. The edges of the bone are finely serrated and fitted together like the pieces of an intricate jig-saw puzzle.

In an infant there is a soft area where the frontal and parietal bones join, which does not ossify until the child is about eighteen months old. This is called the *anterior fontanelle*. It is the easiest site to take the pulse of an infant as the pulsation of the blood vessels can be felt through the soft membrane. There is a

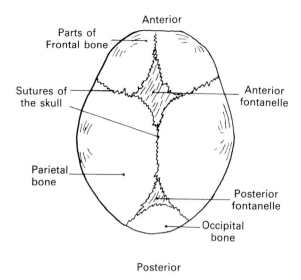

Fig. 2.20 The skull in early infancy—fontanelles

similar fontanelle at the back of the skull but this ossifies in the first few weeks of life. These soft areas allow the skull to be moulded during the birth.

The sinuses of the skull

The sinuses of the skull are spaces containing air in the frontal, ethmoid and sphenoid bones and also in the maxilla. These spaces communicate with the nose. They help in the production of the voice and lighten the skull. Spread of infection from the nose or throat to these spaces results in *sinusitis*.

THE THORAX OR THORACIC CAGE

The thorax is the superior cavity of the trunk. At the back are the twelve thoracic vertebrae to which are attached twelve pairs of ribs. The ribs form the lateral and anterior walls of the thorax and are attached by cartilage to the sternum. The ribs and the sternum are flat bones which form a cage protecting the heart and lungs.

The sternum

The Sternum is the breast bone. It lies just under the skin and can be easily felt. It is shaped like a dagger and has three parts, the *manubrium* or handle, the *body* or blade and the *xiphoid* process or point. The manubrium and body give attachment to the clavicle and ribs.

The sternum is a very light bone, being comprised mainly of cancellous tissue. A *sternal marrow puncture* is a procedure in which a wide bore needle is passed through the thin layer of compact bone in order to remove a specimen of marrow from the cancellous bone. This is done in certain types of blood disorders to examine the maturity of the blood cells.

The heart lies immediately behind the body of the sternum. *External cardiac massage* is a means of stimulating the heart to beat again after it has stopped. This is done by rhythmically pressing on the sternum and so massaging the heart until it starts to beat on its own. When performing cardiac massage it is important to place the 'heel' of the hand on the lower third of the body of the sternum and not on the xiphoid process, as this might easily be broken off by the pressure exerted.

The ribs

There are twelve pairs of ribs, seven pairs of true ribs and five pairs of false ribs. A rib is a flat curved bone attached posteriorly to the thoracic vertebrae by the *head* and *tubercle*. The shaft curves backwards then forwards and is attached to the sternum by pieces of cartilage called the *costal cartilages*. These cartilages give a spring to the thorax which helps to prevent fractures occurring as a result of a blow on the chest. However, if the blow is sufficiently violent the ribs will fracture and this injury may then be complicated by damage to the lungs by the fractured ribs.

The last five pairs of ribs are the so-called false ribs. The eighth, ninth and tenth pairs have costal cartilages, but they are attached only indirectly to the sternum by means of the

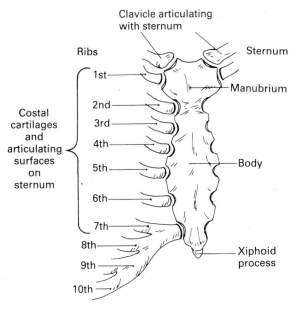

Fig. 2.21   The sternum

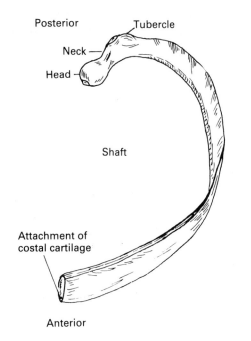

Fig. 2.22   A rib (left)

seventh costal cartilage. The last two pairs have no cartilage. They are the *floating ribs* and are embedded in muscle tissue.

The anterior and posterior attachments of the ribs are freely movable, allowing easy up-

wards and outwards movements of the chest on breathing.

THE SHOULDER GIRDLE

The shoulder girdle consists of two clavicles or collar bones and two scapulae or shoulder blades. These bones form an incomplete girdle round the upper part of the thorax. The function of the shoulder girdle is to give the upper limb a greater range of movement.

The clavicle

The clavicle is an S-shaped bone. It can be felt along the whole of its length if you run your finger from the prominence where it is attached to the sternum to the point of the shoulder where it has an attachment to the spine of the scapula.

The function of this bone is to act as a strut to hold the shoulders back. If it is broken, usually as a result of a fall on the outstretched hand, the whole shoulder falls forwards and downwards. The application of a figure-of-eight bandage or harness aims at bracing the shoulder back into position until the bone heals.

The scapula

The scapula is a flat bone. The word means a digging tool. It has a large flat blade and a han-

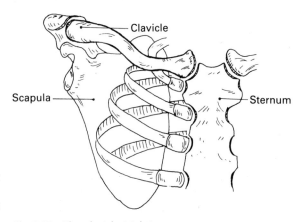

Fig. 2.23   The clavicle (right)

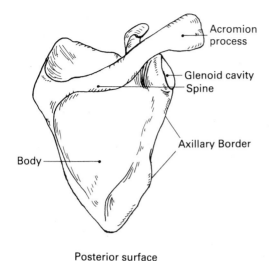

Fig. 2.24 The scapula (right)

dle which projects from the back. The blade of the scapula is the body of the bone. It is separated from the ribs by muscle and moves on the back of the thorax giving the shrugging movements of the shoulders.

The body of the scapula is triangular in shape and therefore has three angles and three sides or borders. The lateral border forms one of the boundaries of the space under the arm called the *axilla*. At the top of this border is a shallow saucer-shaped surface called the *glenoid cavity*. This is the surface which articulates with the head of the humerus to form the shoulder joint.

Projecting from the posterior surface is the *spine*. This lies just under the skin and can be felt along its whole length from the middle of the back to where it unites with the clavicle at the *acromion process* above the shoulder joint.

THE UPPER LIMBS

Each upper limb consists of:
    a humerus in the upper arm
    a radius and ulna in the forearm
    eight carpal bones of the wrist
    five metacarpals and fourteen phalanges of the hand and fingers

The humerus

The humerus is a long bone. The upper extremity has a rounded *head* which articulates with the glenoid cavity of the scapula. Lateral to the head is the greater *tubercle* (tuberosity), a rough process for the attachment of muscles. This process together with the spine of the scapula form pressure points when the patient is nursed in the lateral position.

Below the upper extremity the bone narrows to form the shaft. This narrow part is called the surgical *neck*. In injuries to the shoulder this is a site which is sometimes fractured. Winding round the back of the shaft is the *radial nerve* which supplies the muscles which pull up the wrist and straighten the fingers. Careless handling of an unconscious patient or incorrect use of crutches may damage this nerve and result in a dropped wrist. When an unconscious patient is placed on a theatre table or trolley the nurse must make sure that the arms are well supported and do

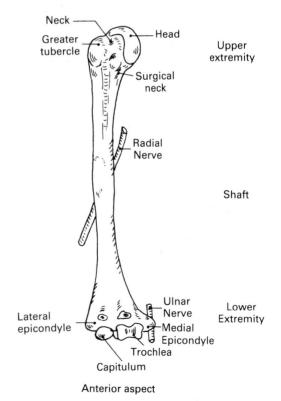

Fig. 2.25 The humerus (right)

not hang over the edge where the radial nerve would be compressed between the edge of the table and the humerus.

The lower extremity of the humerus is broader and flatter than the upper extremity. It has two articular surfaces forming the elbow joint. The pulley-shaped *trochlea* for the ulna and the rounded *capitulum* for the radius. There are two projections on either side called *epicondyles*. The skin over these projections requires regular attention if the patient is bed-ridden because it is liable to become sore from rubbing against the sheets. The *ulnar nerve* winds round the back of the medial epicondyle where it can be rolled against the bone. If sufficient pressure is exerted the sensation of tingling can be felt in the ring and little finger, hence the term 'funny bone'.

The bones of the forearm

The radius

The radius is the lateral bone of the forearm. In the anatomical position it is the bone in line

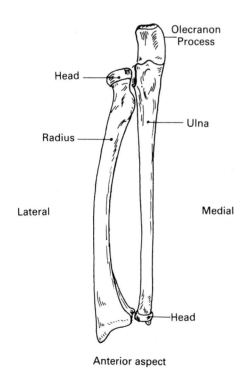

Fig. 2.26 The radius and ulna (right)

(labels on figure)
Olecranon Process
Head
Radius
Ulna
Lateral
Medial
Head
Anterior aspect

with the thumb. It is a long bone with a round button-shaped upper extremity called the *head*. The head articulates with the humerus to form part of the elbow joint and also with the ulna to give the rotating movements of the forearm.

The lower extremity is larger and flatter than the upper extremity. It articulates with two of the carpal bones to form the wrist joint and also with the lower extremity of the ulna. The *radial artery* passes over the front just below the thumb. At this point it can be compressed against the bone. This is the most convenient site at which to feel the pulse.

The ulna

The ulna is the medial bone of the forearm. It is a long bone with a claw-shaped upper extremity which articulates with the humerus and radius. The upper part of the claw is the *olecranon process* which forms the point of the elbow. This is another site where the skin quickly becomes red from rubbing on the sheets.

The lower extremity of the ulna consists of a small rounded *head* which can be seen at the back of the wrist in line with the little finger. The head articulates with the carpus and the radius.

The bones of the hand

The skeleton of the hand consists of three parts:
the carpus—the bones of the wrist
the metacarpals—the bones in the palm
the phalanges—the bones of the fingers

The carpus

The carpus consists of eight short carpal bones arranged roughly in two rows of four. The proximal row articulates with the radius and ulna and the distal row with the metacarpals. There is free gliding movement between each bone but because of their shape and arrangement a strong unit is formed which can take the weight of the body.

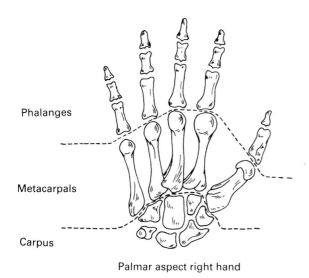

Phalanges

Metacarpals

Carpus

Palmar aspect right hand

Fig. 2.27   The bones of the hand

The metacarpals

The metacarpals are long bones. There are five of them in the palm of the hand. Their rounded heads form the *knuckles*.

The phalanges

The phalanges are minature long bones. There are fourteen in all, three in each finger and two in the thumb.

THE PELVIS

The pelvic girdle

The pelvic girdle consists of the two large irregular bones called the innominate bones. These bones articulate with the sacrum posteriorly to form the pelvic cavity. As this cavity contains the organs of reproduction, the formation of the female pelvis differs from that of the male. The male pelvis is smaller, narrower and more funnel shaped than the female pelvis which is large, wide and cylindrical in shape.

The innominate bone

Three bones fuse together during childhood to form the innominate bone. The upper part

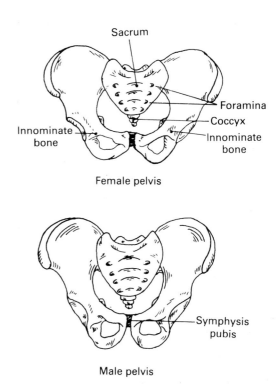

Sacrum
Foramina
Coccyx
Innominate bone
Innominate bone

Female pelvis

Symphysis pubis

Male pelvis

Fig. 2.28   The pelvic girdle

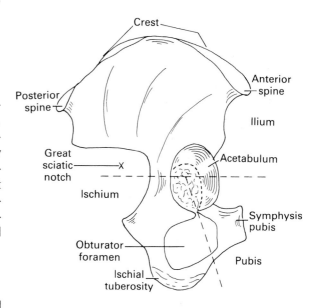

Crest
Anterior spine
Posterior spine
Ilium
Great sciatic notch
Acetabulum
Ischium
Symphysis pubis
Obturator foramen
Pubis
Ischial tuberosity

Fig. 2.29   The innominate bone (right)

is flat and the rest irregular. The three bones are the ilium, the ischium, and the pubis

The ilium is the flat upper part which has the powerful hip muscles of the buttocks attached to it. At the top of the bone is a thick curved *crest* which ends in sharp *spines* anteriorly and posteriorly. This crest can be felt just below the waist. Below the posterior spine is the great sciatic notch where the *sciatic nerve* comes out of the pelvis into the buttock.

The ischium is the lower posterior portion of the bone. It has a large prominence called the *ischial tuberosity* which takes the weight of the body when seated. These tuberosities are protected by small sacs of fluid called *bursae* which act as water cushions. It is therefore possible to maintain the correct sitting position for a considerable period of time without friction occurring between skin and bone. These points require care and attention when the patient is thin and confined to a wheel chair. He must be taught to sit correctly, and, if his arms are strong enough, to raise himself up once every five to ten minutes. This will change his position slightly so that the same area of skin is not continually being compressed between chair and bone.

The pubis is the thin anterior portion of the innominate bone. The two pubic bones join in front at the *symphysis pubis* which is just anterior to the bladder. In fractures of the pelvis one of the dangers is injury to this organ.

All three parts of the innominate bone unite at the cup-shaped *acetabulum*. This is the socket into which the head of the femur fits to form the hip joint. Below the acetabulum is a large hole called the *obturator foramen*. In addition to providing passage for a nerve going to the lower limb this hole reduces the weight of the pelvic girdle.

THE LOWER LIMBS

Each lower limb consists of:-
    a femur—the thigh bone
    a tibia and a fibula—the leg bones
    the tarsal bones of the ankle

the metatarsals and phalanges of the foot and toes

The femur

The femur is the longest and strongest bone in the body. The upper extremity has a rounded *head* which fits into the acetabulum to form the ball and socket hip joint. Just below the head is the narrow *neck* which in the elderly can fracture as a result of very trivial injuries. Lateral to the neck is the greater *trochanter* which, with the lesser trochanter below, gives attachment to many muscles. The greater trochanter takes most of the pressure when the patient is nursed in the lateral position. Not only must the skin over this area receive great care but the patient must be turned from one side to the other every two to three hours to allow the circulation to be restored to the skin.

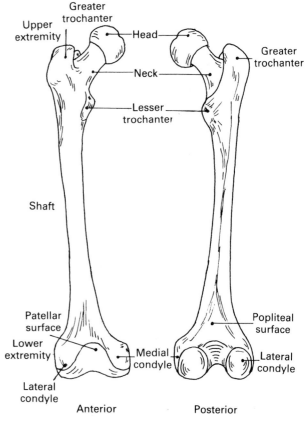

Fig. 2.30 The femur (right)

The shaft is long and curved slightly forwards. It ends in two rounded *condyles* which join with the tibia to form the knee joint. In the lateral position the condyles must be kept apart by the use of pillows otherwise the medial condyle of one knee will rub on the other. Above the condyles anteriorly is the smooth *patellar surface* and posteriorly the triangular-shaped *popliteal surface*. The popliteal space is the area behind the knee through which blood vessels and nerves pass to the leg.

Pressure on a blood vessel slows the circulation and tends to make the blood clot. The resulting thrombosis is a serious post-operative complication which is encouraged by placing a pillow under the patient's knees. The patient must therefore be assisted in moving around in bed and in exercising his legs. If the sitting position has to be maintained, this should be done by using a foot rest or an adjustable bed, never a knee pillow.

The patella

The patella is a sesamoid bone, a type of short bone developed in the tendon of a muscle. It is triangular in shape and forms the knee cap. It takes the weight in the kneeling position. Like the ischial tuberosity, it is protected from friction by a small bursa.

The patellae are pressure points in either the prone or supine positions. In the former they must be protected from rubbing on the sheets. It the latter a bedcage must be used to support the weight of the bedclothes, especially if flexion deformities of the knees are present.

The tibia

The tibia is the medial bone of the leg. It is thicker than the fibula and, of the two bones of the leg, is the one which takes the weight. It is a long bone with an expanded upper extremity which consists of two prominent *condyles* which articulate with the femoral condyles to form the knee joint.

The shaft is triangular in section with a very superficial anterior border. This is the *tibial crest* or shin. The lower extremity helps to

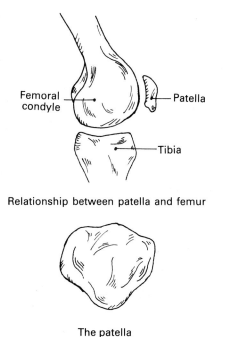

Relationship between patella and femur

The patella

Fig. 2.31 The patella (right)

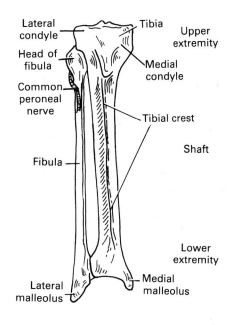

Anterior aspect

Fig. 2.32 Tibia and fibula (right)

form the ankle joint with the fibula and one of the tarsal bones. The prominent bony projection on the inner border is the *medial malleolus*. Like the medial condyles of the femur the malleoli, unless protected, will rub on each other when the patient is in the lateral position.

The fibula

The fibula is the lateral bone of the leg. The upper extremity of this bone is a rounded *head* which can be felt on the outside of the knee slightly towards the back. The important *common peroneal nerve* winds round this prominence. This nerve is easily damaged by pressure and, as it supplies the muscles which pull up the foot, injury to it will cause drop foot, a deformity similar to that caused by tight bedclothes. When applying a knee bandage, care must be taken to see that the head of the fibula is padded and that the bandage is not too tight. It should be fastened in front, not at the side, and knots should be avoided. A hard pad or pillow must never be placed under the knee, and the area should always be protected from the pressure of leg splints.

The lower extremity of the fibula is the *lateral malleolus*. It is the outer bone of the ankle and may be subjected to pressure and friction from the bedclothes.

The bones of the foot

The skeleton of the foot consists of three parts:
  the tarsus—the bones of the posterior half of the foot
  the metatarsals—the bones of the anterior half of the foot
  the phalanges—the bones of the toes

The tarsus

The tarsus consists of seven short bones, the tarsal bones, which take the weight of the body in the standing position. Two of these

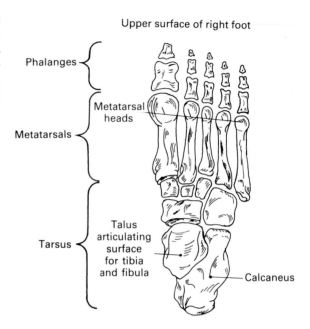

Fig. 2.33 The bones of the foot

bones are larger than the others. The *talus* is the third bone involved in the formation of the ankle joint. The *calcaneus* is the largest bone. It projects backwards and forms the heel.

The metatarsals

The heads of the five metatarsals form the 'ball' of the foot.

The phalanges

There are fourteen phalanges forming the toes. As in the fingers, each toe has three phalanges except for the big toe which has only two.

The arches of the foot

The bones of the foot are arranged in such a way that they form three arches: two lengthwise and one across the front of the foot. These arches give the foot its spring, and if they fall, the resulting gait will be ungainly and

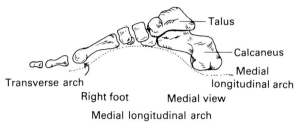

Talus

Calcaneus

Medial longitudinal arch

Transverse arch

Right foot   Medial view

Medial longitudinal arch

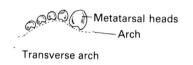

Metatarsal heads

Arch

Transverse arch

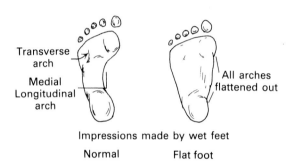

Transverse arch

Medial Longitudinal arch

All arches flattened out

Impressions made by wet feet

Normal   Flat foot

Fig. 2.34 The arches of the foot

the feet painful. There are many causes of flat feet, amongst them the habitual wearing of badly made slip-on shoes. Patients who have been confined to bed for a long period and young people who have just left school to take up a job which requires long periods of standing, are particularly in need of good supporting shoes.

The pressure areas of the foot

The pressure areas of the foot are the toes and the heels. The bedclothes press on the toes and the heels rub against the sheet. A bedcage will take the weight off the toes, and pressure can be removed from the heels by the use of small soft pillows.

The skeletal system questions

Diagrams—questions 36–86

36–40   Diagram of a long bone
   A. Red bone marrow
   B. Compact bone tissue
   C. Hyaline cartilage
   D. Medullary canal
   E. Periosteum

36
37
38
39
40

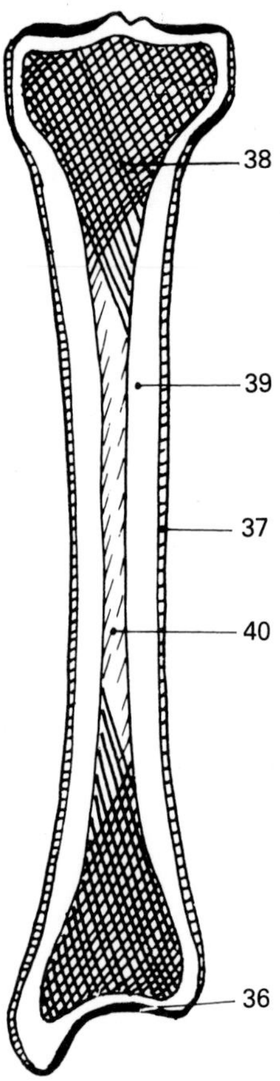

41–44. Diagram of a growing bone

A. Epiphysis	41
B. Diaphysis	42
C. Epiphyseal cartilage	43
D. Primary centre of ossification	44

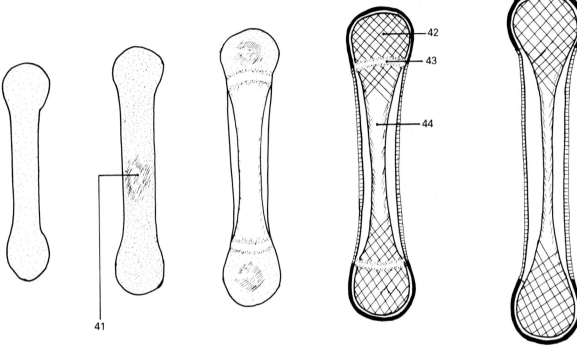
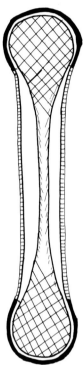

45–50. A vertebra

A. Body	45
B. Lamina	46
C. Pedicle	47
D. Neural arch	48
E. Spinous process	49
F. Vertebral foramen	50

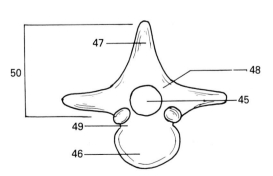

51–57. **The skull**

A. Temporal bone	51
B. Frontal bone	52
C. Lacrymal bone	53
D. Maxilla	54
E. Mandible	55
F. Nasal bones	56
G. Zygomatic bone	57

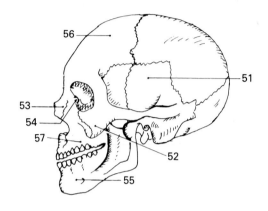

58–61. **The scapula**

A. Acromion process	58
B. Inferior angle	59
C. Glenoid cavity	60
D. Spine	61

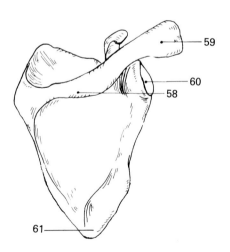

62–66. **The humerus**
- A. Capitulum
- B. Head
- C. Lateral epicondyle
- D. Surgical neck
- E. Trochlea

	62
	63
	64
	65
	66

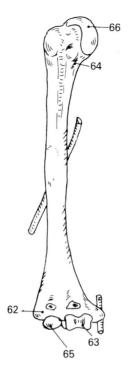

ANTERIOR ASPECT

67–70. **The radius and ulna**
- A. Distal radio-ulnar joint
- B. Head of radius
- C. Head of ulna
- D. Olecranon process

	67
	68
	69
	70

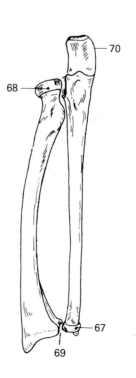

71–75. **The innominate bone**

    A. Acetabulum

    B. Ischial tuberosity

    C. Iliac crest

    D. Great sciatic notch

    E. Symphysis pubis

71	
72	
73	
74	
75	

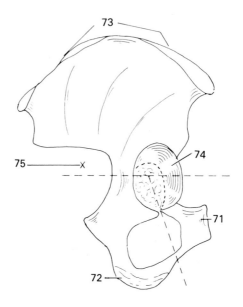

76–80. **The femur**

    A. Head

    B. Neck

    C. Greater trochanter

    D. Medial condyle

    E. Patellar surface

76	
77	
78	
79	
80	

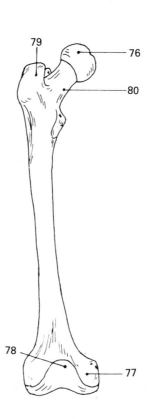

81–86. The tibia, fibula and foot

A. Calcaneus	81
B. Head of fibula	82
C. Medial condyle of tibia	83
D. Medial malleolus	84
E. Talus	85
F. Tibial crest	86

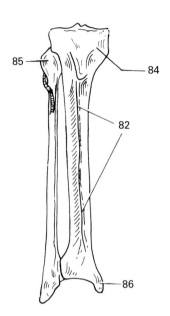

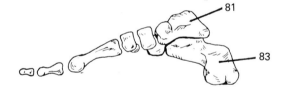

Questions 87–95 are of the multiple choice type

87. **Which one of the following statements describes the term proximal?**
    A. Away from the midline
    B. Near the midline
    C. Nearest to the body
    D. Palm down.

87

88. **Which one of the following describes a foramen in a bone? It is :**
    A. a groove
    B. a hole
    C. a notch
    D. a smooth surface.

88

89. **Living bone tissue consists of one of the following:**
    A. 5% water
    B. 25% water
    C. 90% solids
    D. 50% solids.

89

90. **The number of lumbar vertebrae is :**
    A. 12
    B. 7
    C. 5
    D. 4.

90

91. **Which one of the following statements describes the parietal bones? They :**
    A. contain the foramen magnum
    B. form the orbits
    C. are part of the face
    D. are part of the cranium.

91

92. **The mastoid process is a part of the following bones. Which one?**
    A. Frontal
    B. Occipital
    C. Sphenoid
    D. Temporal.

92

93. **The nerve of smell passes through one of the following bones. Which one?**
    A. Ethmoid
    B. Frontal
    C. Nasal
    D. Sphenoid.

93

94. The ribs are classified as:

A. Long bones
B. Flat bones
C. Short bones
D. Irregular bones.

95. The bones of the thumb are classified as :

A. Long bones
B. Flat bones
C. Short bones
D. Irregular bones.

Questions 96–111 are of the true/false type

	T	F

96–99. The growth of bone tissue is influenced by :
    96. the amount of calcium in the diet
    97. the amount of iron in the diet
    98. the amount of vitamin B in the diet
    99. the endocrine glands.

100–103. The term supine means :
    100. lying face down
    101. lying face up
    102. palm down
    103. palm up.

104–107. The cervical curve is :
    101. a primary curve
    105. a secondary curve
    106. concave backwards
    107. concave forwards.

108–111. The Xiphoid process is :
    108. a part of one of the bones of the face
    109. the attachment of the 11th rib
    110. part of the sternum
    111. anterior to the heart.

Questions 112–120 are of the matching items type

112–114. **From the list on the left select the anatomical part which forms the structure on the right.**

A. Acromion process	112. Funny bone	112
B. Greater trochanter	113. Knuckles	113
C. Heads of the metacarpals	114. Point of elbow.	114
D. Medial epicondyle		
E. Olecranon process		

115–117. **From the list on the left select the anatomical part which is formed by the structure on the right.**

A. Calcaneus	115. Heel	115
B. Patella	116. Knee cap	116
C. Talus	117. Shin.	117
D. Tibial crest		
E. Tibial condyle		

118–120. **From the list on the left select the site where damage might result in the development of the condition on the right.**

A. Lateral aspect of the knee	118. Dropped wrist	118
B. Medial malleolus	119. Dropped foot	119
C. Pelvis	120. Paraplegia.	120
D. Shaft of humerus		
E. Vertebral column		

3

The joints and the muscles

Having studied the bones of the skeleton, we must now find out how they are joined together. The next step will be to clothe the skeleton with muscles. These give the body its contours and ensure that the appropriate movements can occur.

JOINTS OR ARTICULATIONS

A joint is a junction between two or more bones. It is classified into one of the following three groups, according to its structure and movement:

fibrous or immovable
cartilagenous or slightly movable
synovial or freely movable

Fibrous joints

In a fibrous joint the opposing edges of the bones are joined together by fibrous tissue. This fixes the joint so that no movement is possible. The sutures of the skull are examples of this type of joint.

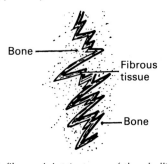

Fig. 3.1 A fibrous joint (sutures of the skull)

Cartilagenous joints

The cartilagenous joints have pads of white fibrocartilage between the bones. This cartilage can be compressed to give slight movement. Examples are the joints between the bodies of the vertebrae.

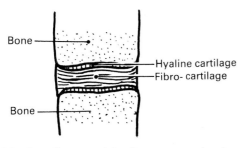

Bone

Hyaline cartilage
Fibro- cartilage

Bone

Fig. 3.2 A cartilagenous joint (between vertebrae)

Synovial joints

The main synovial joints are the joints of the limbs and the joints between the limbs and the shoulder and pelvic girdles. The name means like an egg (syn—like, ovum—an egg). Each synovial joint is lubricated by a sticky clear fluid like the white of an egg. This type of joint is more complicated than the others and requires further study.

A typical synovial joint

If you examine a synovial joint you will see that the ends of the bones fit together fairly accurately. These joining surfaces are covered with *hyaline cartilage* and are held together by a cuff of white fibrous tissue called the *capsule*. The capsule has a smooth lining of a specialised tissue called *synovial membrane*. The membrane secretes the viscid fluid which acts as a lubricant and allows the surfaces to move on each other without friction. Synovial membrane covers every structure inside the joint capsule except the hyaline cartilage. It also forms bursae and sheaths for the tendons of those muscles which have long tendons passing over several joints, for example, the muscles which move the fingers.

Each joint is strengthened by the presence of *ligaments*. Some lie inside the joint but most of them are outside the capsule. These ligaments act as strong ties holding the bones together. If a ligament is torn, it may result in a dislocation or displacement of the joint surfaces. A sprain is the condition which results when some of the fibres are torn but the ligament remains intact.

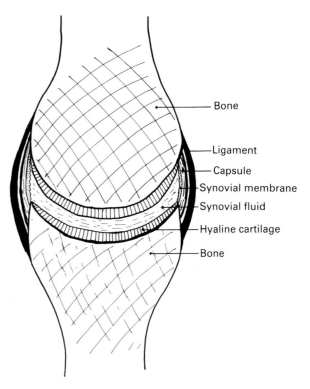

Bone

Ligament
Capsule
Synovial membrane
Synovial fluid
Hyaline cartilage
Bone

Fig. 3.3 A synovial joint

Certain terms are used to describe the movements of the synovial joints. These are:
gliding is sliding
flexion is bending
extension is straightening
rotation is turning
adduction is moving towards the midline
abduction is moving away from the midline
inversion is turning the foot inwards
eversion is turning the foot outwards
circumduction is a movement which involves flexion, extension, adduction, abduction and rotation
The synovial joints are classified according to their shape and movements.

Type of Joint	Movement
Gliding or plane	sliding
Hinge	flexion and extension
Pivot	rotation
Condylar and saddle	flexion, extension, adduction and abduction
Ball and socket	flexion, extension, adduction, abduction and rotation

Gliding joints

Gliding joints consist of small flat surfaces which slide on each other. The joints between the neural arches of the vertebrae are examples of gliding joints.

Hinge joints

The elbow, the ankle, the interphalangeal joints and the knee are all hinge joints.

The movements of the elbow joint are flexion and extension. Rotation of the forearm occurs at the superior radio-ulnar joint which is closely associated with the elbow joint (See Fig. 2–26).

The movements of the ankle joint are *dorsiflexion*, which is carrying the top of the foot up towards the leg, and *plantarflexion*, which is pointing the toes. The movements of *inversion* and *eversion* do not occur at the ankle. They are produced by the bones of the tarsus gliding on each other. The interphalangeal joints are the joints of the fingers and toes which can be curled up (flexion) and straightened out (extension).

The knee joint is much more complicated, as it has to support the weight of the body in addition to being freely movable. It is not a true hinge joint as slight rotation is possible when the knee is flexed. This joint has intracapsular structures which add to its strength. Two ligaments cross each other in the centre of the knee joining the tibia to the femur. These are the *cruciate ligaments*. If you look at the shape of the articular surfaces, you will see that the rounded condyles of the femur sit on the flat surfaces on the condyles of the tibia. Two crescent-shaped cartilages act as

wedges, deepening the surface of the tibia to receive the femoral condyles. These are the *menisci*, the cartilages which get torn in certain injuries to the knee. The outside of the capsule is strengthened by ligaments and also by the powerful *quadriceps muscle* which forms the front of the knee joint and has the patella in its tendon.

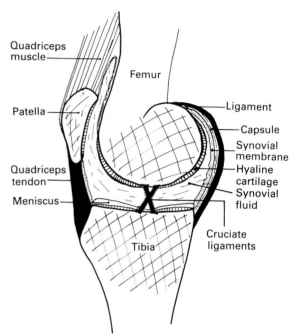

Fig. 3.4 A knee joint (Lateral view)

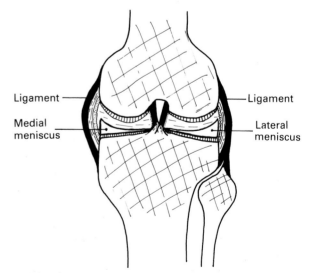

Fig. 3.5 A knee joint showing the menisci (Anterior view)

Pivot joints

The radio-ulnar and the atlanto-axial joints are pivot joints. The atlanto-axial joint has already been described. It permits the rotating or shaking movements of the head.

The radio-ulnar joints allow the radius to rotate over the ulna, giving the movements of *pronation* and *supination*. There are two radio-ulnar joints in each forearm. The proximal joint is just below the elbow joint and the distal joint is just above the wrist joint.

Condylar joints

The temporomandibular, the wrist, the metacarpophalangeal and the metatarsophalangeal joints are condylar joints. The movements of the temporomandibular joints produce the opening, closing and chewing movements of the jaw.

The movements of the *wrist* joint are flexion, which is called *palmar flexion*, and extension, called *dorsiflexion*. Adduction or ulnar deviation and abduction or radial deviation are also possible. A patient with rheumatoid arthritis is quite likely to have a degree of ulnar deviation contraction of the wrist and fingers, resulting in an obvious deformity.

The metacarpophalangeal and the metatarsophalangeal joints allow flexion and extension and when the fingers and toes are extended, adduction and abduction.

The carpometacarpal joint of the thumb is a *saddle joint*. It has the additional movements of rotation and circumduction and can be *opposed* to the other fingers for grasping movements.

Ball and socket joints

The hip and shoulder joints are ball and socket joints. Together with the knee joint they are classified as atypical synovial joints.

All the basic structures of a synovial joint are present in the *shoulder joint*, but a glance at the scapula and humerus will remind you that the glenoid cavity is oval and very shallow and the head of the humerus is round. This arrangement provides unrestricted movement, but creates a joint which is potentially unstable.

To ensure stability the following additional structures are present in the shoulder joint.

Surrounding the glenoid cavity and deepening it is a rim of fibrocartilage (the labrum), which helps to hold the head of the humerus against the scapula more securely.

One tendon of the biceps muscle passes from the scapula to the humerus through the joint capsule and helps to steady the joint in various movements.

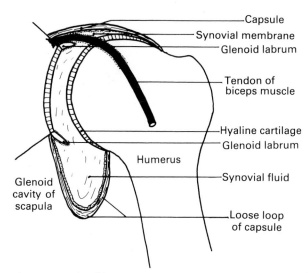

Fig. 3.6a   A shoulder joint

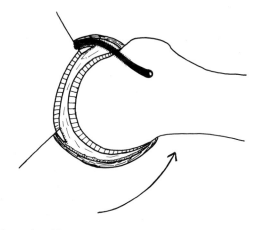

Fig. 3.6b   A shoulder joint in abduction

The capsule is very lax to allow for the wide range of movement of the shoulder joint, especially abduction. The joint can be dislocated by a fall, blow or twist when the arm is abducted, usually during sporting activities.

The ball and socket structure is more obvious in the *hip joint* than in the shoulder joint. The hip joint, although capable of all movements, is a very stable joint. The ball-shaped head of the femur articulates with the cup-shaped acetabulum of the innominate bone. The head of the femur is covered with hyaline cartilage except for a small depression. This is where the apex of a triangular-shaped ligament is attached. The base of this ligament is attached to the lower margin of the acetabulum and carries an extra blood supply to the head of the femur. The acetabulum is only partially covered with hyaline cartilage and it is deepened by a rim of fibrocartilage called the *labrum*. The great strength of this joint is dependent upon the external ligaments of the capsule, especially the anterior *iliofemoral ligament* which is the strongest ligament in the body. Traumatic dislocation of this joint is uncommon.

Synovial joints are meant to be moved, and fixation for any reason will result in progressive stiffness and pain. The joint capsule will tighten and contractures will form. A contracture of a joint may produce a very distressing and disabling deformity. Arthritis, which is inflammation of a joint, is a painful condition. The patient resists movement of his joints and will adopt the most comfortable position even if this produces crippling joint contractures. One reason why the nurse must learn about the joints is to enable her to assist the physiotherapist in keeping painful joints mobile, and so preventing deformities.

THE MUSCLES

The muscles form the flesh of the body. They are made of voluntary or striped muscle tissue and are attached to the bones by tendons. If you take a piece of lean meat and tease it out you will see that it consists of bundles of threadlike structures. These threads are the muscle cells. They vary in length and are called muscle *fibres*. Each fibre has horizontal, light and dark stripes and contains many nuclei. They are arranged in bundles called *fasciculi*. Each fasciculus is surrounded by areolar tissue. A muscle consists of many such bundles enveloped in a further sheet of areolar tissue

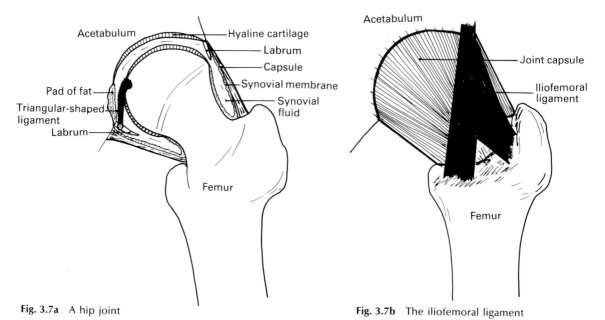

Fig. 3.7a A hip joint

Fig. 3.7b The iliofemoral ligament

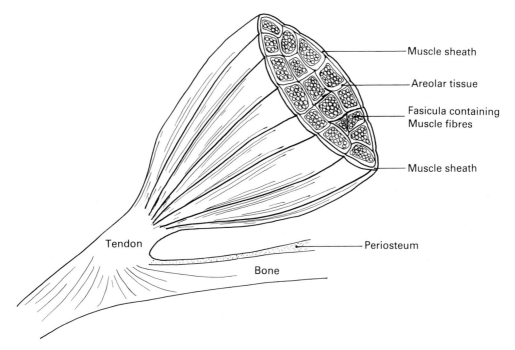

Fig. 3.8 Muscle structure

which is continuous with the *tendon*, attaching it to bone.

Each muscle fibre can, when stimulated, contract. This means that it gets shorter and thicker. As the muscle passes over one or more joints this contraction will pull one bone towards the other thus producing movement at the joint. If a powerful movement is required, as for example when lifting a heavy weight, many more fibres will contract than would be necessary for lifting a pencil. The type of movement depends on the position and shape of the muscles and the type of joint it crosses.

A muscle must possess an adequate blood supply and a nerve supply before it can contract. From the blood the muscle receives **glucose** and **oxygen**. Glucose comes from carbohydrate foods and oxygen from the air breathed into the lungs. The nerve supplies the impulse which starts off a series of chemical changes involving the glucose and oxygen. These changes release the energy which makes the muscles contract.

In a petrol-driven engine the sparking plug ignites the mixture of petrol and air. This re-

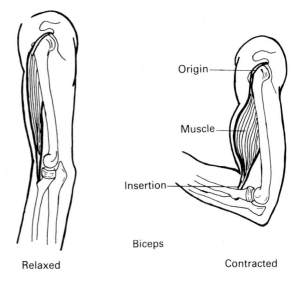

Fig. 3.9 Muscle action

leases the energy which makes the machinery work and the wheels move. As a result of this combustion the engine becomes hot and there must be some means of keeping it cool. In many cars this is achieved by having a radiator which must be kept full of water. As long as the engine is running, waste gases, mainly carbon dioxide, are being released into the atmosphere.

Now compare the human body with this engine. Food replaces the petrol, glucose being the body's fuel. The glucose can be stored in the muscle, just as petrol is stored in the petrol tank. When movement is required, the carbohydrate is broken down, oxygen is carried to the muscles in the blood stream and a series of chemical changes occur which release energy and produce heat. The energy makes the muscle contract and the heat helps to keep the body temperature at 37°C.

In any activity requiring excessive use of muscles more glucose is required and the individual must take deeper breaths to get more oxygen to the muscles. More heat is produced but the body temperature does not go up because the sweat glands in the skin become more active. Sweat consists mainly of water. This water evaporates from the skin surface and in so doing uses up excess body heat. It also means that the body loses more water so the individual gets thirsty. This can be corrected by taking a drink.

The engine which drives the car has an exhaust system which gets rid of the waste products of combustion. The body must also rid itself of waste. The waste produced by muscle action is *carbon dioxide* and water. These are conveyed by the blood to the lungs and breathed out, although some of the water is also excreted by the skin, the urinary bladder and the bowel.

Just as a car will refuse to move if not supplied with petrol or if the battery requires to be recharged, so will the muscles become inactive if anything interferes with the blood and nerve supply. Damage to, or blockage of, a blood vessel will interfere with fuel and oxygen supply. An overtight bandage, particularly a plaster one, is enough to do this. If left uncorrected for too long it will deprive the muscle of its blood supply and the muscle will die. If the brain, spinal cord or nerves are damaged or diseased, the controlled passage to the muscle of the nerve impulse will be prevented and the muscle will be paralysed. If the injury or disease is in the brain or spinal cord, the

muscles become *spastic*. Spastic paralysis occurs when the muscles cannot relax because the controlling influence from the brain has been cut off. They are contracted and hard and will pull the affected joints into abnormal positions.

If the nerves are diseased or damaged, the muscles lose their tone and become *flaccid*. Muscle *tone* is a state of slight contraction which is maintained in normal muscle tissue, keeping it ready for action. When it loses its tone, the muscle becomes soft and flabby and cannot contract. This accounts for the grotesque deformities which sometimes occurred in patients who suffered from poliomyelites.

Nurses must learn how to handle and support affected muscles and how to maintain body posture so that these deformities are prevented. This is the reason for learning about the joints and muscles. It is not necessary to study all the muscles of the body but knowledge of some of the following is important in nursing.

THE MUSCLES OF THE HEAD, NECK AND TRUNK

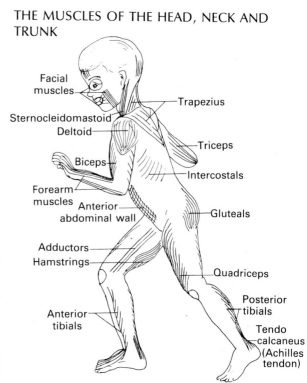

Fig. 3.10 Superficial muscle groups

The muscles of the head

There are many small muscles in the head and only two movable joints. The muscles which move the temporomandibular joints are the muscles of mastication (chewing). The other muscles are the muscles of the face. They are attached to the skin, the lips and to the eyes. These are the muscles of facial expression.

The muscles of the neck

There are two main groups of muscles in the neck. At the back are the two extensor muscles each called *trapezius*, and in front the flexor muscles, each called *sternocleidomastoid.* The two trapezius muscles receive their name from their combined shape (both muscles together form a four-sided figure). The sternocleidomastoid muscles receive their name from their attachments. If you work out the attachments of the sternocleidomastoid muscles you will see that when they both contract together they will flex the head on the chest, but that one muscle acting on its own will pull the mastoid process round towards the sternum and rotate the head. The tendon which attaches the muscle to the stationary bone, in this case the sternum, is called the origin of the muscle. The tendon attached to the bone which moves is the tendon of insertion.

The muscles of the thorax

The thoracic muscles are the *intercostal muscles* and the *diaphragm*. The intercostals lie between the ribs. When they contract they raise the ribs upwards and tilt them outwards, and this movement increases the size of the thoracic cavity on inspiration. The diaphragm is a dome-shaped sheet of muscle between the thorax and the abdomen. It is attached to the lower ribs, the lumbar vertebrae and the sternum and forms a floor for the thoracic cavity. When it contracts, it flattens out and makes the chest deeper. Both the diaphragm and the intercostals are important muscles of respiration (see Ch. 5).

The muscles of the abdominal wall

The anterior abdominal wall consists of four layers of flat muscles which have several functions. These muscles maintain the positions of the abdominal organs. Should they weaken in any way, the result might be the displacement of an organ or part of an organ. This is called a *hernia* or rupture. The abdominal muscles also help in movements of the spine, in breathing, coughing, sneezing and in emptying the bladder (micturition) and the bowel (defaecation).

When a patient is being prepared for abdominal examination, his bladder should be empty and he should lie flat on his back with only one pillow. This ensures complete relaxation of the muscles and allows the doctor to palpate the organs.

Coughing is caused by irritation of the respiratory passages. When you cough the abdominal muscles contract, forcing the abdominal organs against the diaphragm, and this pushes more air out of the lungs in an effort to expel the irritating material. Patients, who have had abdominal operations, try to avoid coughing because any sudden muscular contraction results in a spasm of severe pain. The post-operative care given by the physiotherapist involves teaching the patient to cough whilst supporting the wound. If he does not cough up the mucus produced by the irritated lining of the lungs, pneumonia may develop.

The muscles of the pelvic floor

The *levator ani* muscles are flat muscles attached to the pelvis. They unite with each

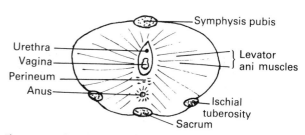

Fig. 3.11 Pelvic floor

other to form the pelvic floor which helps to support the pelvic organs. There are three openings through the female pelvic floor. The anterior opening is the *urethral* orifice, leading from the bladder. The *vaginal* orifice, leading to the uterus, is the middle opening and the posterior opening forms the *anus*, which is the exit from the bowel. The male pelvic floor has only the urethral and anal openings. The area between the anus and the anterior openings is the *perineum*. Weakness of the perineum may result in a prolapse of the pelvic organs.

THE MUSCLES OF THE UPPER LIMB

The muscles of the shoulder joint

There are several muscles surrounding the shoulder joint, the largest and most superficial being the *deltoid* muscle. This is a large thick triangular muscle which arises from the shoulder girdle and is inserted into the shaft of the humerus just where the radial nerve winds round the bone (Fig. 1.25). This muscle abducts the shoulder. It is sometimes used as a site for intramuscular injections. In this case the arm must be removed from the sleeve and the injection given well up towards the shoulder where there is no danger of damaging the nerve.

The muscles of the upper arm

The muscles of the upper arm lie between the shoulder and the elbow, and their main action is on the elbow joint.

In front is the *biceps* muscle. It is a powerful flexor of the elbow and a supinator of the forearm. Its tendon of insertion into the radius can be felt in front of the elbow. This tendon is just lateral to the brachial artery and may be used as a guide to the positioning of the stethoscope when blood pressure is being recorded.

The posterior muscle of the upper arm is the *triceps* muscle which extends the elbow.

The muscles of the forearm and hand

The anterior muscles of the forearm have tendons which cross the wrist, and some of them

extend to the tips of the fingers. These muscles *palmarflex* the wrist and *flex* the fingers. The posterior muscles have the opposite action. They extend or *dorsiflex* the wrist and *extend* the fingers.

An important group of muscles in the hand forms the ball of the thumb. These are the *thenar* muscles which allow the thumb to be opposed to the fingers, thus producing the important grasping movements necessary for most manual skills.

THE MUSCLES OF THE LOWER LIMB

The muscles of the hip

The muscles which form the buttock are the *gluteal* muscles. They abduct, rotate and extend the hip. They play an important part in maintaining the upright position of the body.

As these muscles are bulky they are frequently used as a site for intramuscular injections. The large *sciatic* nerve passes through the gluteal muscles on its way down into the lower limb. It lies towards the midline of the body and in the lower part of the buttock. It is important to avoid this nerve when giving

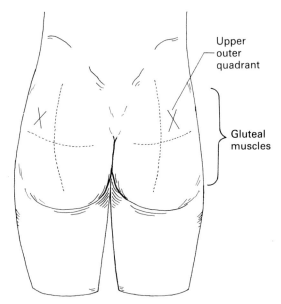

Fig. 3.12 Site for intramuscular injections into the buttock

an injection into the buttock, as injury to the sciatic nerve will produce almost complete paralysis of the limb. The safest site for injection into the buttock is the upper and outer quadrant.

The *psoas* muscle, which flexes the hip, arises from the lumbar vertebrae. It passes in front of the hip through the pelvis to be inserted into the femur.

The muscles of the thigh

There are three groups of muscles in the thigh. The *adductor* muscles of the hip lie medially, in front is the *quadriceps* muscle and at the back lie the **hamstring** muscles.

The quadriceps femoris is the great extensor of the knee. It arises from the shaft of the femur and is inserted into the tibia by the patellar tendon. This muscle is important in maintaining the upright position and in walking. It should be kept exercised by all patients especially those who are suffering from affections of the knee joint.

The hamstring muscles are three muscles at the back of the thigh which flex the knee. In diseases of the knee joint the tendons of these muscles may become permanently contracted. This produces a flexion contracture of the knee, when the knee cannot be straightened.

The safest site for intramuscular injections is perhaps the lateral aspect of the thigh, as no large nerves or blood vessels pass through this region.

The muscles of the leg and foot

The muscles in front of the leg, the *anterior tibial* muscles, have long tendons which pass over the ankle joint and are inserted into the toes. These are the dorsiflexors of the ankle and the extensors of the toes.

The **posterior tibial** muscles form the bulk of the calf. They are inserted into the calcaneus by a very thick strong tendon sometimes called the *tendon* of *Achilles*. These muscles plantarflex the ankle and raise the heel off the ground when walking.

The muscles of the leg also flex the toes, invert and evert the foot and support the arches.

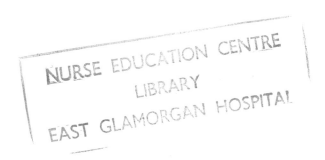

The joints and the muscles questions

Diagrams—Questions 121–137

121–124. A synovial joint

    A. Capsule

    B. Synovial membrane

    C. Ligaments

    D. Hyaline cartilage.

121

122

123

124

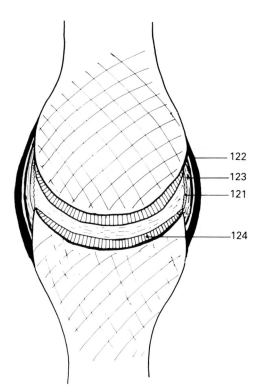

125–128. The pelvic floor

    A. Anus

    B. Perineum

    C. Urethra

    D. Vagina

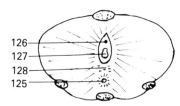

125

126

127

128

129–137. Muscles of the skeleton

A. Biceps	129
B. Trapezius	130
C. Triceps	131
D. Intercostals	132
E. Deltoid	133
F. Quadriceps	134
G. Hamstrings	135
H. Gluteals	136
I. Sternocleidomastoid.	137

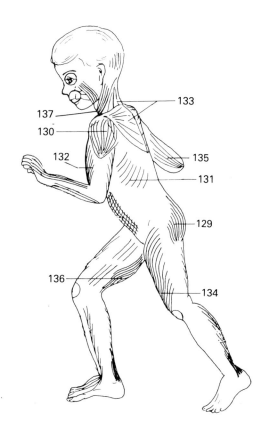

Questions 138–145 are of the multiple choice type

138. **Which one of the following statements describes adduction?**
    A. Bending forwards
    B. Moving away from the midline
    C. Moving towards the midline
    D. Turning inwards.

139. **The anterior fontanelle ossifies at :**
    A. 1 month
    B. 10 months
    C. 18 months
    D. 24 months.

140. **Which one of the following is a hinge joint?**
    A. Ankle
    B. Metacarpophalangeal joint
    C. Temperomandibular joint
    D. Wrist.

141. **Which one of the following movements is possible at the elbow joint?**
    A. Dorsiflexion
    B. Extension
    C. Inversion
    D. Rotation.

142. **The radio-ulnar joints are :**
    A. gliding joints
    B. hinge joints
    C. pivot joints
    D. saddle joints.

143. **The wrist joint is the joint between one of the following groups of bone. Which one?**
    A. The carpus and the metacarpus
    B. The distal extremities of the radius and ulna
    C. The radius and ulna and the proximal carpal bones
    D. The radius and ulna and the distal carpal bones.

144. **Which one of the following is a waste product of muscle contraction?**
    A. Carbon monoxide
    B. Glucose
    C. Oxygen
    D. Water.

145. Paralysis is the condition which results from :
  A. Dead muscle tissue
  B. Diseased muscle tissue
  C. Muscle deprived of its nerve supply
  D. Muscle deprived of its blood supply.

Questions 146–165 are of the true/false type   **T** | **F**

146–149. A muscle fibre :

146. is its cell
147. is striped longitudinally
148. has more than one nucleus
149. is the covering of the muscle.

150–153. The diaphragm :

150. is a dome-shaped muscle
151. is a muscle of respiration
152. rises when it contracts
153. separates the thorax from the abdomen.

154–157. The deltoid muscle :

154. lies over the shoulder joint
155. adducts the upper limb
156. raises the shoulder girdle
157. connects the upper limb to the shoulder girdle.

158–161. The gluteal muscles :

158. cover the sciatic nerve
159. flex the hip
160. keep the trunk upright in walking
161. rotate the hip.

162–165. The quadriceps muscle :

162. extends the hip
163. extends the knee
164. is the medial muscle of the thigh
165. is inserted into the tibia.

Questions 166–174 are of the matching items type

166–168. From the list on the left select the movement which can occur at each joint listed on the right.

A. Plantarflexion	166. Radio-ulnar joints	166
B. Eversion	167. Tarsal joints	167
C. Supination	168. Wrist joint.	168
D. Ulnar deviation		

169–171. From the list on the left select the anatomical structure which is part of each joint on the right.

A. Acetabulum	169. Knee	169
B. Glenoid cavity	170. Hip	170
C. Lamina	171. Shoulder.	171
D. Obturator foramen		
E. Femoral condyle		

172–174. From the list on the left select a movement which is produced by each muscle listed on the right.

A. Abduction of the shoulder	172. Intercostals	172
B. Extension of the neck	173. Sternocleidomastoid	173
C. Rotation of the head	174. Trapezius.	174
D. Mastication		
E. Inspiration		

4

The circulatory system

The circulatory system consists of the heart, the blood vessels and the blood. It is the means by which the food and oxygen are conveyed from the digestive tract and lungs to the body cells. The waste products are also conveyed by this system from the cells to the organs which excrete them. The heart acts as a pump keeping the blood circulating through the blood vessels.

Some harmful substances, which are dangerous if present in the body, enter a secondary circulation called the lymphatic system, where they may be destroyed before reaching the blood stream. This system consists of lymphatic vessels, nodes and ducts. A clear yellowish fluid called lymph circulates through these vessels. The spleen, an abdominal organ, is also associated with this system.

The circulatory and lymphatic systems communicate with each other and will be studied together.

THE HEART

The heart is a hollow cone-shaped organ which lies between the lungs in the space in the middle of the thorax called the *mediastinum*. It is tilted slightly more towards the left side than to the right. It is situated behind the sternum and in front of the oesophagus and the large blood vessels. The base of the heart lies uppermost to the right side of the chest at the level of the second rib. The apex is on the left side in contact with the diaphragm at the level of the fifth and sixth ribs (see Fig.1 21).

The myocardium

The wall of the heart is made of cardiac muscle tissue and is called the myocardium. This tissue also forms a *septum*, dividing the organ into a right and left side. Cardiac muscle tissue is capable of contracting on its own. It is stimulated to contract by small areas of specialised tissue dispersed in the wall. This system is called the 'pace maker'.

The outside of the heart is covered by fibrous tissue and the inside is lined with epithelium. The epithelial tissue forms valves which divide the organ into two upper and two lower chambers. The chambers are called the *atria* and the *ventricles*. The right and left atria are uppermost at the base of the heart and the right and left ventricles are below at the apex. The blood flows from the atria to the ventricles from where it is pumped round the body.

The myocardium is thinner in the atria which receive blood from the blood vessels, and thicker in the ventricles which push the blood out into the circulation. The function of the myocardium is to act as a pump. It contracts and squeezes the blood out, and when it relaxes it allows the heart to fill up with blood again. Any change in the rate, force or rhythm of the contractions can be detected by the nurse when she feels the pulse.

The pericardium

The outer covering of the heart is called the pericardium. It is a sac of fibrous tissue lined with a second sac of epithelial tissue. The outer fibrous sac is continuous with the covering of the large blood vessels which enter and leave the heart at its base. It is protective in function and because it is tough it prevents the heart from overdistending. The inner sac secretes a thin lubricating fluid called serum. This serum prevents friction as the heart contracts and relaxes within the fibrous pericardium. Should the pericardium become inflamed, the tissues will rub on each other causing pain. This rubbing can be heard if the sounds of the heart are listened to with a stethoscope.

The endocardium

The endocardium is made of squamous epithelium and forms a smooth lining for the blood to flow over. It is continuous with the lining of the blood vessels. The smooth surface prevents clots forming in the blood.

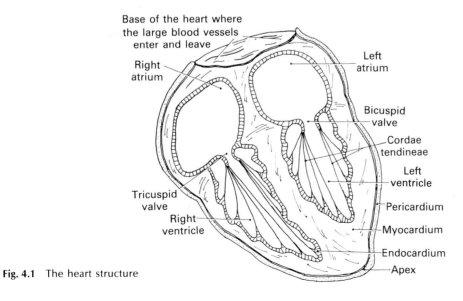

Base of the heart where the large blood vessels enter and leave

Right atrium

Left atrium

Bicuspid valve

Cordae tendineae

Left ventricle

Tricuspid valve

Pericardium

Right ventricle

Myocardium

Endocardium

Apex

Fig. 4.1   The heart structure

Blood will clot readily if it is in contact with a rough surface.

Double folds of endocardium form the valves which divide the atria from the ventricles and prevent the blood from flowing in the wrong direction. The *atrio-ventricular valve* on the right side has three flaps or cusps and is called the *tricuspid valve*. The valve on the left side has two cusps. This *bicuspid valve* is sometimes called the *mitral valve.*

These valves open and close with the flow of the blood. They are attached to the ventricle walls by fibrous cords (*chordae tendineae*) which prevent the valves from turning inside out.

In endocarditis or valvular disease of the heart, the valves may leak or the opening may become so small that insufficient blood gets through. The result of valvular disease in a patient is slowing down of the circulation and an accumulation of excess fluid in the tissues and in the lungs. It is this excess fluid in the tissue which results in the swelling (*oedema*) of the ankles and the breathlessness seen in patients suffering from valvular disease of the heart.

THE BLOOD VESSELS

There are three types of blood vessels:
    arteries which carry blood away from the heart
    capillaries which connect the arteries to the veins
    veins which return the blood to the heart.

The arteries

The arteries leave the heart at the right and left ventricles where they are very large. They branch again and again, getting smaller and thinner and spreading out to every part of the body. The smallest arteries are called *arterioles*. Eventually, these vessels become so small they cannot be seen without a microscope. The arterioles have now become capillaries.

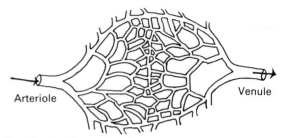

Fig. 4.2 Capillary network

The capillaries

The capillaries are minute vessels which form a network throughout the tissues. They eventually join up to form small veins called *venules*.

The veins

The venules join other venules until veins are formed. The largest veins enter the heart at the right and left atria.

THE STRUCTURE OF THE BLOOD VESSELS

The arteries and veins are constructed in a similar way to the heart. They are muscular tubes with a protective covering and a smooth lining. The muscle coat (*tunica media*) is plain involuntary muscle tissue which is supplied by nerves from the autonomic nervous system (see Ch. 9). This tissue can contract and relax, varying the size of the vessel and depending on the amount of blood required by the tissues it supplies. The muscular walls also contain elastic tissue which allows the vessel to stretch and recoil depending on the amount of blood it contains. There is more elastic tissue in the large arteries than in the small arteries, and there is very little in the veins. The veins have much thinner and softer walls than the arteries: they collapse when cut. Blood will flow from cut veins, but it spurts from cut arteries which retain their shape.

The fibrous covering of the vessels (*tunica adventitia*) is protective in function. The epithelial lining (*tunica intima*) is continuous with the endocardium. It forms valves in the large veins of the limbs where it prevents back-flow of the blood as it travels up against gravity.

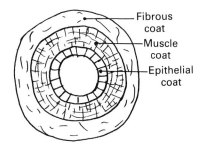

Fig. 4.3 Transverse section of an artery

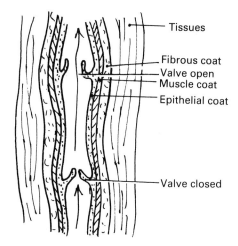

Fig. 4.4 Longitudinal section of a vein

Valves are also present where the large arteries leave the heart.

The walls of the capillaries are continuous with the lining of the arterioles and the venules. They are composed of a single layer of epithelial cells which is thin enough to allow water and nutrients to pass through from the blood to the tissue fluid. The capillaries form a vast network in all the tissues of the body.

Arteriosclerosis is a hardening or narrowing of the muscular wall of an artery, limiting the flow of blood to the part it supplies. This is often the lower limb and can cause severe pain on walking. The pain is due to oxygen starvation of the tissues.

An *aneurysm* is a weak part in the vessel wall which dilates and may burst, causing severe haemorrhage.

An *infarct* is an area of dead tissue. This is often the result of a blocked artery which pre-

vents oxygen from reaching the tissues. When arterial blockage occurs in the myocardium, it causes death of part of the heart muscle (cardiac infarct) and may result in cardiac arrest.

THE CIRCULATION OF THE BLOOD

When we talk about the circulation we mean the passage of the blood from the heart via the arteries to the capillaries and back to the heart via the veins. We will be considering the circulation as four separate systems but each system communicates with the others.

The coronary circulation

The heart itself is the first organ to receive a blood supply. Two important arteries branch from the aorta just as it leaves the left ventricle. These are the *coronary arteries*. These arteries divide and become arterioles and then capillaries. The capillaries join to form venules and veins. The coronary veins drain into a channel called the *coronary sinus* which lies in the wall of the right atrium, the chamber which receives the venous blood. This system of blood vessels is called the coronary circulation and is the means by which the wall of the heart is nourished.

A *coronary thrombosis* is the sudden blocking of a coronary artery by a clot. This is a common cause of sudden death. If the blockage is incomplete, the patient may suffer from severe pain in the region of the heart and down the left arm. This condition is called *angina pectoris*.

The general or systemic circulation

The general circulation consists of the arteries and veins which carry the blood from the left ventricle round the body and back to the right atrium.

The aorta

The blood leaving the left ventricle of the heart passes through the aortic valve into the

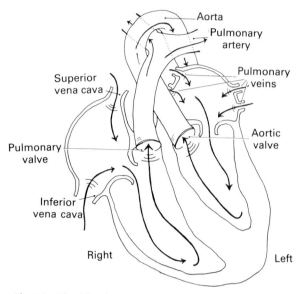

Fig. 4.5 The blood vessels of the heart

aorta. This is the largest artery in the body. The aorta passes upwards then arches over the base of the heart to lie at the back. It passes down through the thorax posteriorly, through an opening in the diaphragm where it enters the abdomen.

The circulation to the upper limb

Leaving the arch of the aorta, where it lies at the base of the neck, are two *subclavian* arteries. These pass into the *axillae* and down the upper arm where they are renamed the *brachial* arteries. The brachial artery is the one which, in First Aid, can be compressed against the humerus to arrest bleeding following an injury to the forearm or hand.

The brachial artery divides in front of the elbow to form the *radial* and *ulnar* arteries. These lie in the lateral and medial sides of the forearm and enter the hand by passing over the wrist. In the hand they become the *palmar* and *digital* arteries. The radial artery can be felt pulsating at the base of the thumb where it lies on top of the radius. This is the most common site for feeling the pulse.

The blood returns from the hand by the veins which lie beside the arteries, sharing their names. The *subclavian* veins join with the

veins of the head to form the *brachio-cephalic* veins. These in turn join to form the superior *vena cava* which enters the right atrium (see Fig. 4.5)

The circulation to the head and neck

The right and left common carotid arteries which lie in the neck are branches of the arch of the aorta. These arteries divide and become the *internal* and *external carotid* arteries. The internal carotid arteries enter the skull and supply the brain. The external carotids divide to supply the face and scalp. Two of their branches can be felt pulsating; the *temporal* in front of the ears and the *facial* arteries in front of the angles of the jaw.

Blood returns from the head and neck by the *jugular* veins which join up with the right and left subclavian veins (see Fig. 4.9).

The circulation in the thorax

The thoracic aorta is the part of the aorta which lies behind the heart. This large artery gives off branches which supply the chest wall, part of the lungs and the oesophagus. Blood from these parts is returned to the heart by veins which join the *superior vena cava*.

The circulation in the abdomen

The abdominal aorta is the continuation of the thoracic aorta which passes through the back of the diaphragm and continues down through the abdomen. It lies in front of the vertebrae, to the level of the 4th lumbar vertebra, where it divides to form the right and left *common iliac* arteries. The abdominal aorta provides branches to the abdominal organs. There are two *phrenic* arteries which supply blood to the diaphragm, the *renal* arteries which supply the kidneys, and the *ovarian* and *testicular* arteries which supply the reproductive organs.

Single arteries supply the other organs. The *hepatic* and *splenic* arteries go to the liver and the spleen respectively. The *gastric* artery sup-

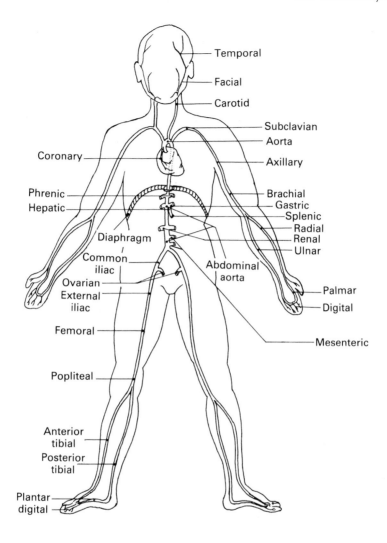

Temporal
Facial
Carotid
Subclavian
Aorta
Axillary
Coronary
Brachial
Gastric
Splenic
Radial
Renal
Ulnar
Phrenic
Hepatic
Diaphragm
Common iliac
Abdominal aorta
Ovarian
External iliac
Palmar
Digital
Femoral
Mesenteric
Popliteal
Anterior tibial
Posterior tibial
Plantar digital

Fig. 4.6 The arteries

plies the stomach, and the *superior* and *inferior mesenteric* arteries carry the blood supply to the bowel.

Veins from the reproductive organs, the kidneys, the liver and the diaphragm enter the *inferior vena cava*. This large vein is formed by the junction of the two common iliac veins which bring blood from the lower limbs. This vein lies at the back of the abdomen to the right of the aorta. It passes through the centre of the diaphragm and enters the heart at the right atrium.

The circulation to the lower limbs

The common iliac arteries divide in the pelvis to form the *internal* and *external iliac* arteries. The internal iliac arteries supply the pelvic organs.

The external iliac arteries pass out of the pelvis into the thighs where they change their names to the *femoral* arteries. In the groin, where these arteries lie on the rim of the pelvis, they can be compressed to arrest bleeding in injuries to the lower limb.

The femoral artery passes round to the back of the knee to become the *popliteal* artery. This artery divides to form the *anterior* and *posterior tibial* arteries which supply the leg and become the *plantar* and *digital* arteries of the foot.

The veins in the lower limbs lie alongside the arteries and have the same names. These are called the deep veins. There is, however, a second set of veins lying just under the skin. These *superficial veins* join the deep vein at the knee and in the groin. They are not supported by surrounding muscles and may become varicosed. *Varicosed veins* have defective valves. As a result the return of venous blood to the heart against gravity is sluggish, the veins dilate and the legs become swollen and painful. The skin nutrition of the legs is impaired and ulcers may develop. Varicose ulcers are very slow to heal.

There are also superficial veins in the upper limbs. These veins are readily seen at the bend of the elbow and at the wrist, and are easily accessible when blood has to be withdrawn or intravenous injections given. These superficial veins do not possess many valves as gravity plays a big part in returning blood from the hand to the heart. For the same reason, they do not become varicosed.

The pulmonary circulation

An important group of vessels carries venous blood containing excess carbon dioxide from the heart to the lungs. In the lungs the carbon dioxide is excreted by expiration and the blood becomes reoxygenated before being returned to the heart and then into the systemic circulation. (see Ch. 5)

The *pulmonary artery* leaves the right ventricle and divides into two branches, one to each lung. Blood is returned to the left atrium by the four *pulmonary veins*, two from each lung (See Fig. 4.5).

The portal circulation

The portal circulation carries blood containing nutrients from the stomach, spleen and bowel to the *liver* (see Ch. 6). The gastric vein, the splenic vein and the mesenteric veins all unite to form the large *portal vein* which enters the liver.

THE BLOOD

Blood is a very active tissue. It carries nutrients, oxygen, hormones, waste products and antibodies from one organ to another. It connects the different parts of the body and is therefore described as a connective tissue. It has a fluid matrix in which cells float. The average individual has about five to six litres of blood circulating.

Everyone knows that blood is a warm, red, sticky and salty fluid. If blood is withdrawn from an individual's vein and is allowed to stand in a test-tube, the red part falls to the bottom and a clear yellowish fluid is left above. The blood is now divided into a solid part and a fluid part. The fluid part is called *plasma*; and the solid part consists of the cells or *blood corpuscles*.

The plasma

About 55% of the blood volume is plasma. This is mainly water with certain substances dissolved in it, some of which come from the food which we digest.

1. *Nutrients*

Glucose from carbohydrate foods. Examples are potatoes and sugar.

Amino acids from protein foods. Examples are meat and fish.

Fats from such foods as milk and butter.

Vitamins from all foods.

2. *Mineral salts*

These have many uses and help to maintain the slight alkalinity of the blood. Examples are sodium chloride and sodium bicarbonate, as well as small amounts of potassium, calcium, magnesium, phosphates, copper and iron.

3. *Waste products*

These are mainly carbon dioxide and urea.

4. *Plasma proteins*
Albumen which exerts an osmotic force and makes the blood sticky.
5. *Clotting substances*
These are prothrombin and fibrinogen.
6. *Antibodies*
7. *Hormones*
These are secretions of the endocrine glands.

The blood cells

There are three types of blood cells:
red blood corpuscles or *erythrocytes*
white blood corpuscles or *leucocytes*
platelets or *thrombocytes*.

Erythrocytes

These corpuscles give the blood its colour. They make up about 99% of the total number of blood cells. They are usually described as biconcave (thin in the middle and thick round the edges), nonnuclear discs. There are about five million in one cubic millimetre of blood in men, and slightly less in women. They tend to adhere to each other and, under the microscope, appear as piles of cells. These erythrocytes can squeeze through the finest capillary.

Each cell is made of *haemoglobin*, a substance which has an affinity for oxygen. When the erythrocytes reach the capillaries which surround the air sacs in the lungs, the haemoglobin combines with oxygen and transports it to all the tissue cells. Erythrocytes carrying oxygen (forming *oxyhaemoglobin*) are bright red, but when they have given the oxygen up to the cells they become bluish red in colour. The blood in the arteries is, therefore, bright red and in the veins it is bluish.

Haemoglobin is a compound of protein and iron. These substances cannot form mature corpuscles unless *vitamin B$_{12}$* is present. Vitamin B$_{12}$ (cyanocobalamin) is found in certain foods. Before it can be absorbed, a substance, secreted by the stomach, called the *intrinsic factor* must be present. If this factor is absent, the red blood corpuscles do not develop properly and the individual suffers from *pernicious anaemia*.

The word *anaemia* means a deficiency of haemoglobin. This may be due to a lack of red blood cells or to a deficiency in their haemoglobin content. The most common type of anaemia is *iron deficiency* anaemia, which may be due to loss of blood or lack of iron in the diet. This type of anaemia is very common in women.

Erythrocytes are developed in the red bone marrow. When they reach maturity they pass into the blood stream where they convey oxygen to the tissue cells. This oxygen carrying function of the erythrocytes is of vital importance. Each corpuscle lives for about four months. It is then destroyed by the spleen and broken down into its component parts. The iron is recycled and used by the bone marrow to manufacture more haemoglobin. The protein part is carried to the liver where it forms one of the ingredients of *bile*.

As each cell dies it is replaced. If many cells are lost, as in the case of haemorrhage, then the bone marrow produces more.

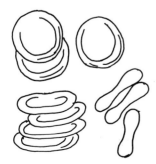

Fig. 4.7 Erythrocytes

Leucocytes

The white blood corpuscles are the scavengers of the body. They have what is called a phagocytic action. They travel to an area of tissue which has become infected by micro-organisms, surround the organisms, destroy and digest them. They can be compared to an army going abroad to fight the enemy. However, if the organisms are strong, the result can be destruction of the affected tissue and the cells.

This is how *pus* is formed. It consists of dead tissue cells, leucocytes and micro-organisms.

There are several different types of *leucocyte* formed in the bone marrow. They are larger than the erythrocytes, much fewer in number and all possess a nucleus. Some of the leucocytes have very fine granules in the protoplasm and are called *granulocytes*. Granulocytes can squeeze through the capillary wall to attack the invading micro-organisms. Others have no granules and are called *lymphocytes*. Lymphocytes are to be found in the blood, the *tonsils*, the *spleen* and the *lymph nodes*. These corpuscles destroy micro-organisms and play a part in the formation of antibodies.

Fig. 4.8 A selection of leucocytes

Antibodies destroy any substance which is foreign to the body. These foreign substances are called *antigens*. The presence of an antigen stimulates the production of more lymphocytes. When kidney or other organ transplantations are undertaken, the body recognises the presence of foreign material. Drugs must be given to suppress the action of the leucocytes so that the new organ will not be rejected by the body. The patient being given these *immunosuppressive* drugs must therefore be protected from any exposure to infection.

Leukaemia is a malignant disease affecting the white blood corpuscles. They increase in number, are immature and crowd out the healthy cells. An acute type of leukaemia occurs in children, and if untreated is quickly fatal.

Thrombocytes

These are small oval discs present in the blood in large numbers. They do not possess a nu-

cleus and are smaller than the other cells. They also come from the bone marrow.

Thrombocytes are sticky. When the wall of a blood vessel is damaged they stick together and plug up the hole until a clot is formed.

The clotting mechanism. The thrombocytes liberate a substance called thromboplastin which acts on the *prothrombin* and *calcium* in the blood producing *thrombin*. Thrombin acts on the *fibrinogen* in the plasma and *fibrin* is formed. The threads of fibrin form a network in which the blood cells are trapped. This is the clot which will occlude the opening in the blood vessel and prevent bleeding (see Table 4.1).

Table 4.1 The mechanism of clotting

Thrombocytes		Blood plasma		
Thromboplastin	+	Calcium and prothrombin	=	Thrombin
Thrombin	+	Fibrinogen	=	Fibrin
Fibrin	+	Blood cells	=	Clot

If you study the formation of a clot in a test tube you will see that it shrinks, and as it does so a clear yellowish fluid appears. This is serum and it consists of plasma minus the clotting substances. If a flowing specimen of blood is required, sodium citrate is added to the specimen because this chemical prevents the formation of the clot.

The application of a rough dressing will speed up the rate at which a clot will form in a wound. A smooth oily dressing will slow it down.

A clot forming in an intact vessel is called a *thrombus*; it is commonly caused by a narrowing of, or damage to, the blood vessel wall. This is usually accompanied by a sluggish circulation. The presence of a thrombus in the deep veins of the calf is a common complication of bed rest. This is one of the reasons why early ambulation and leg exercises should follow surgery whenever possible.

An *embolus* is a solid body or an air bubble carried in the circulation. Part of a thrombus may become detached and travel in the blood stream to the heart where it may block the pulmonary artery. This is a *pulmonary em-*

bolism; it is a complication of deep venous thrombosis and is usually fatal.

Present in the blood is an anticoagulant called *heparin* which prevents clotting. Usually, there is just enough to keep the blood flowing. Heparin can be given intravenously in the treatment of thrombosis. When a patient is receiving anticoagulant therapy, the nurse must be very observant because there is always a danger of bleeding.

Blood groups

When a patient is to have a blood transfusion a specimen of his blood is sent to the haematology department to be grouped and crossmatched. Before blood is transfused it must be checked very carefully to ensure that the patient receives blood which is compatible with his own. He must receive blood of the correct group.

In the walls of the red blood corpuscles there are antigens and in the plasma antibodies. Remember that antibodies destroy antigens. The antigens are called *agglutinogens* and are classified A, B, AB or O. The antibodies are called *agglutinins* and are classfied Anti-A and Anti-B.

Individuals are divided into four blood groups A, B, AB and O. If a person's blood belongs to group A, his antigen is A but his antibody is Anti-B. If he is transfused with blood group B which contains Anti-A antibodies the donor cells will clump together (agglutinate). This blood is incompatible and the patient will become very ill. His temperature will rise, he may become jaundiced and the clumped cells may block the kidney tubules causing renal failure.

An individual with blood group AB has no agglutinins (antibodies) and can therefore receive blood from any other group. He is known as a universal recipient.

An individual with blood group O has Anti-A and Anti-B agglutinins (antibodies) but no agglutinogens (antigens). There are, therefore, no antigens to be destroyed so he can give his blood to any group. This person is a universal donor.

Crossmatching means taking some of the donor cells together with the recipient's plasma and observing if clumping of the cells occur (see Table 4.2).

Table 4.2

Cell-Antigen	Group Plasma-Antibody	Transfusion Can be transfused with
A	Anti-B	A and O
B	Anti-A	B and O
AB	None	A, B, AB and O
O	Anti-A and Anti-B	O

The rhesus factor

In the blood of threequarters of the world population there is a substance called the Rhesus factor. Those of us who have this factor are said to be Rhesus positive, the others are Rhesus negative. Normally, there are no antibodies in the plasma against the Rhesus factor, but if Rhesus positive blood is given to a Rhesus negative patient Rhesus positive antibodies will appear in the blood. Any subsequent transfusion of Rhesus positive blood might be fatal, as the patient now has antibodies which will act against the transfused cells.

A pregnant woman who is Rhesus negative may be carrying a child who has inherited Rhesus positive blood from its father. A reaction may occur in the blood of this fetus causing destruction of the red cells and jaundice. To prevent severe damage it is sometimes necessary to change the child's blood completely either before or after birth.

THE LYMPHATIC SYSTEM

The lymphatic system consists of an additional set of vessels through which some of the tissue fluid passes before reaching the large veins and entering the blood. This system consists of *lymphatic capillaries, vessels, ducts* and *nodes*. The fluid in the system is called *lymph*.

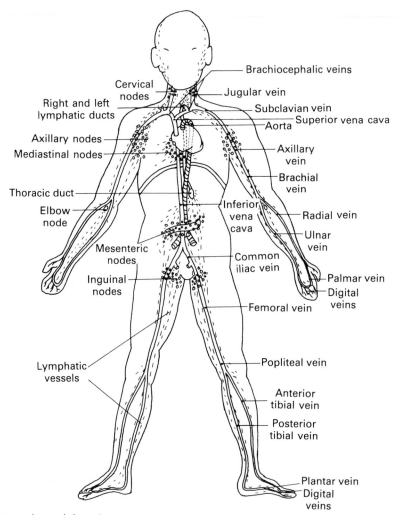

Fig. 4.9 The lymphatic nodes and the veins

Lymphatic capillaries are present in many tissues. They form networks in the tissue spaces but unlike the blood capillaries they start as blind tubes with rounded ends. They are larger than the blood capillaries and more porous, allowing such substances as micro-organisms to pass from the tissue fluid to the lymph (see Fig. 4.10).

The lymphatic vessels are similar in structure to the small veins. They have more valves and these give them a beaded appearance. Several vessels enter one lymphatic node, but the lymph leaves the node by one larger vessel. Eventually, the larger vessels join up to form ducts which are about the size of medium-

sized veins. There are two lymphatic ducts. The *thoracic duct* commences below the diaphragm, passes into the thorax and joins the systemic circulation in the neck at the junction of the left subclavian and jugular veins. The right lymphatic duct is only about 1 cm in length and opens into the junction of the right subclavian and the right jugular veins.

The lymphatic nodes are generally about the size and shape of small beans and are situated at strategic points in the body. They contain lymphocytes and the lymph must pass through one or more of these nodes before it enters the blood stream. The nodes act as filters preventing the passage into the blood of any bacteria, damaged cells or tumour cells which may have passed from damaged tissue into the lymph. The lymphocytes break down these substances but, unfortunately, are not always able to hold back invading organisms or tumour cells.

Until the discovery of antibiotics in the middle of this century a septic finger could be fatal. The virulent organism gained access to the blood and caused blood poisoning or *septicaemia* to develop. The leucocytes were 'on their own' in the fight against the invading organisms. Nothing given by mouth could destroy them without also destroying healthy body cells.

Infection from a sore throat may result in swollen painful 'glands' in the neck which can be palpated easily. These so-called glands are the *cervical lymph nodes* which filter the lymph from the head and neck. A septic finger may cause swelling of the *axillary nodes*, and if lymphatic vessels are inflamed a red streak can be seen on the arm. A septic toe can cause swelling of the *inguinal nodes* which are situated in the groin.

The lymphatic drainage from the breast is into the axillary nodes. When the surgeon is performing a mastectomy for cancer of the breast, he sometimes considers it necessary to remove these lymphatic vessels and nodes.

This is to ensure that all cancer cells which have travelled to the axilla are removed, but it also blocks off the flow of lymph from the arm. This limb may become very oedematous and heavy.

There are lymphatic nodes in the *thorax*, *abdomen* and *pelvis*. These nodes are closely related to the organ they drain. The nodes receiving lymph from the intestines are situated in the *mesentery* which is the covering of the intestines. These nodes become enlarged in infection and tumours of the bowel. The lymphatic drainage of the chest is into the nodes which lie in the *mediastinum*, the space between the lungs in which the heart lies. In city dwellers and cigarette smokers the lymph in these nodes is often black from inhaled dirt and smoke.

The tonsils

There are several other areas of lymphoid tissue in the body. The tonsils form part of a protective ring of tissue at the entrance to the respiratory and digestive tracts. Lymphatic vessels leave the tonsils and enter the cervical nodes.

The spleen

The spleen is a purplish, half-moon shaped organ in the left hypochondriac region of the abdomen. It lies below the diaphragm and behind the lower ribs, and is mainly composed of lymphoid tissue enclosed in an elastic fibrous capsule.

The spleen has several functions. It contains lymphocytes, some of which get into the blood stream to carry out their phagocytic action. It destroys worn out erythrocytes producing bile pigments and iron. It produces antibodies and is capable of providing extra red blood corpuscles in cases of emergency when there is hypoxia. Hypoxia means that there is a diminished amount of oxygen in the tissues. The extra erythrocytes increase the amount of oxygen which can be carried in the blood.

The spleen can only be felt if it is enlarged. Enlargement may occur in a variety of conditions. One of these is acute infection, when the spleen enlarges to meet the increased needs of the body for lymphocytes. The spleen can be removed surgically with few serious effects on the patient, as other tissues in the body take over its functions.

The thymus gland

The thymus gland is a soft, greyish-pink gland which is present in the thorax behind the sternum. It is large in infants and growing children and it reaches its maximum size at puberty. After puberty this gland gradually disappears until in adult life there is only a minute piece of fatty tissue left.

The functions of the thymus are not completely understood but it is necessary for the development of lymphoid tissue in infancy.

A SUMMARY OF THE CIRCULATION

Having studied the structure and function of the various parts of the circulatory system we will now consider the work of the circulation as a whole.

The system is full of blood. There are about five to six litres in the normal individual. The heart beats once every four/fifths of a second, that is about 75 times per minute. The pumping action is stimulated by electrical impulses from the pacemaker (*sinoatrial node*) in the wall of the right atrium. The atria contract and push the blood through the bicuspid and tricuspid valves into the ventricles. The electrical signals now reach the ventricles through a special band of tissue in the septum called the *atrio-ventricular node* or *bundle of His*. This tissue carries the electrical impulses to the walls of the ventricles causing them to contract. The contraction pushes the blood out into the systemic and pulmonary circulations by the aorta and the pulmonary artery. At this stage the atrio-ventricular valves are closed and the aorta and pulmonary valves are open. The muscular walls of the atria and the ventricles then relax and the heart fills up with blood once more.

Venous blood enters the right atrium through the inferior and superior vena cava and arterial blood enters the left atrium by the four pulmonary veins. This is the only part of the circulation where venous blood flows through arteries and arterial blood flows through veins. The blood containing carbon dioxide leaves the right ventricle by the pulmonary artery and travels to the lungs where the interchange of gases takes place. The oxygenated blood then returns to the left artrium by the four pulmonary veins.

The septum of the heart not only divides it into two sides but it separates the arterial blood from the venous blood. Some babies are born with a defect in the septum which allows some of the venous blood to mix with the arterial blood. This contamination of the arterial blood means that it cannot carry the normal amount of oxygen. The baby is blue around the lips and at the fingers and toes. This condition is called *cyanosis*. Because the muscles are not getting enough oxygen the patient will have difficulty in breathing and walking. Fortunately, this 'hole in the heart' condition can be rectified by surgery.

The blood leaves the heart by the large arteries which have elastic walls. As the blood

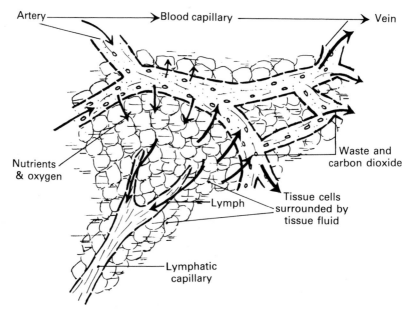

Fig. 4.10 The movement of tissue fluid

is pushed into them these arteries stretch, and when the heart relaxes they recoil. This pushes the blood along into the smaller vessels. Eventually, this arterial blood reaches a network of capillaries. At the arteriole end of this network, water, oxygen and nutrients are pushed through the walls of the capillaries into the tissue fluid by the pressure of the blood. The tissue fluid circulates through the tissues, giving up oxygen and nutrients to the cells and collecting waste products.

There are two routes by which the water and waste can get back into the blood stream. Some of the fluid is sucked through the walls of the capillaries at the venule end by the osmotic force of the albumen in the blood. The rest returns to the blood, having gone through the lymphatic system. If there is an abnormality of the lymphatic vessels or insufficient albumen in the blood, fluid will collect in the tissues. The part becomes swollen and will 'pit' if pressed by the fingers. This condition is called *oedema*.

The blood in the capillaries and the lymph in the lymphatic capillaries must now get back to the heart by the veins and lymphatic vessels. As the heart dilates between each contraction, venous blood is sucked into the right atrium. This is assisted by the action of the diaphragm in deep breathing. Inspiration has a sucking effect on the blood in the inferior vena cava and on the lymph in the thoracic duct. The muscles in the limbs have a similar sucking effect on the veins and lymphatic vessels. When they contract they 'milk' the blood and lymph up towards the heart. The numerous valves prevent back-flow. Gravity plays an important part in returning the blood to the heart from the head and neck, and also from the upper limbs when they are held above the shoulders.

A patient may not be able to move his limbs as a result of pain following an operation or the application of a plaster of Paris cast. The affected limb must be elevated to encourage the return of the blood by gravity. As soon as possible, the patient is encouraged to move his fingers or toes. As this is done by contracting the muscles of the leg and forearm, the improved circulation decreases the swelling and helps to relieve the pain. Deep breathing exercises are also helpful, and the patient should be encouraged to move around in bed until he is able to get up.

BLOOD PRESSURE

The pressure of the blood in the blood vessels is the force which pushes the fluid through the walls of the capillaries. It is therefore important that it is maintained within normal limits.

The greatest force is required to take the oxygen to the brain cells, and they will be the first to suffer as a result of any fall in blood pressure. This is one of the causes of fainting. A low blood pressure also slows the circulation through the skin and makes the patient more prone to pressure sores. Any great rise in blood pressure may result in the capillaries in the brain rupturing and the resulting blood clot damaging the brain tissue. This happens in *cerebral haemorrhage*.

There are several factors which, working together, maintain the blood pressure within normal limits. These are:

the amount of blood circulating (blood volume)

the force with which the heart pumps (cardiac output)

the elasticity of the large arteries

the calibre of the small arterioles (peripheral resistance).

The amount of blood circulating

This will be less in shock and haemorrhage. A badly injured patient or a patient who has had a major operation will have a low blood pressure if untreated. If blood has been lost, as in haemorrhage, this is replaced by whole blood. If the blood volume has been reduced, as in some forms of shock, saline or dextrose solution may be given until the volume of the blood circulating has been returned to normal.

The cardiac output

This depends on the volume of blood which returns to the heart by the veins. If the venous return is poor, the amount of blood leaving the heart is less. Less force is required, the heart beat is weak and the blood pressure is low. Sometimes in the operating theatre, the nurse or medical student in attendance must stand still for long periods of time. The venous return from the lower limbs is inhibited because of gravity and lack of exercise. The heart beat weakens and the blood pressure falls. Add to this the shock of seeing an operation for the first time and you will understand why the new student faints.

The elasticity of the large arteries

This maintains the continuous flow of the blood out to the periphery of the body. As they stretch and recoil they push the blood into the smaller vessels. If the walls of the vessels are hardened, as they may be in old age, the pressure of the blood against the inelastic walls is greater.

The peripheral resistance

This is the state of slight contraction of the muscular walls of the arterioles, producing resistance to the flow of blood. These vessel walls can dilate or contract depending on the amount of blood required by the organ they supply. Heat causes *vasodilation* in the skin and cold causes *vasoconstriction*. When the vessels are dilated the pressure is lower and when they are constricted the pressure is greater. This can be demonstrated by filling a syringe with water. Push the piston and the water flows out. Now add a fine bore needle and the water spurts out with considerable force.

In hot weather or after a hot bath, the arterioles dilate, the skin gets red because there is more blood circulating, but the pressure will be less. The brain gets less oxygen and the individual is less active. On the other hand, cold weather or a cold bath has a stimulating effect.

The skin arterioles are constricted and the blood pressure is increased.

A badly shocked patient has a low blood pressure. This fall in pressure is compensated for by constriction of the arterioles in the skin. This is why the patient's skin looks white and feels cold. It is dangerous to overheat the patient because this will cause vasodilation which will make the skin feel warmer but the heat will lower the blood pressure still further.

THE CARDIAC CYCLE

Blood pressure is recorded by a *sphygmomanometer*. There are always two recordings, one low and the other high. The higher pressure is normally around 110 millimetres of mercury (110 mmHg) and is the pressure in the arteries when the heart is contracted. This period of contraction is called *systole*. Systole lasts for 2/5th of a second. The pressure recorded is called the *systolic* blood pressure. The contraction is followed by a period of rest when the heart fills up with blood. This period also lasts for 2/5th of a second and is called *diastole*. During diastole the heart is not pumping and the pressure is less, usually about 80 mmHg. This is *diastolic* blood pressure. Blood pressure is recorded with the systolic pressure noted above and the diastolic pressure noted below. (110/80 mmHg)

The *cardiac cycle* consists of *systole* plus *diastole* and takes place every 4/5th of a second. The other 1/5th is the beginning of the next cycle. The cycle therefore occurs about 70 times each minute.

The beat of the heart is controlled by electrical impulses from the pacemaker. This electrical activity can be recorded on an *electrocardiograph*. The tracing of one cardiac cycle will appear as shown in Figure 4.11.

The P wave is the period of contraction of the atria, Q, R and S is the contraction of the ventricles and T is the beginning of the period of rest.

A stethoscope is used to listen to the heart beat. This is placed over the apex of the heart and the heart sounds will be heard. These are

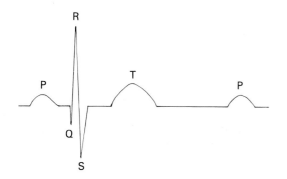

Fig. 4.11 Cardiac cycle

described as 'lubb dup' and are the sounds made by the valves closing.

THE PULSE

The pulse is the beat of the heart as felt at an artery. The pulsation is caused by the stretching of the elastic walls of the arteries during systole when the heart is pushing blood out into the aorta. This wave of distension extends out to the periphery and can be felt where an artery lies over bone. By counting the pulsations a record can be made of the rate at which the heart is beating. At the same time various other pieces of information about the heart and blood vessels can be obtained.

The pulse may be rapid or slow, weak or strong, rhythmical or irregular. These observations will tell you about the state of the heart. A rapid weak pulse may be a sign of internal haemorrhage. The heart beat is weak because the volume of blood going into it is less. It is rapid in order to get the reduced volume of blood round the body. An irregularity in rhythm denotes an irregular heart beat. The time between each beat should be the same but sometimes one beat may be much weaker than others and appears to be 'missed'.

The normal pulse rate changes with the position of the individual. It is quicker when an individual is active and slower when he is at rest. A child has a more rapid pulse than an adult and a woman's pulse is more rapid that a man's. Emotion and exercise increase the pulse rate. A trained athlete, however, has a slow pulse but a much stronger heart beat.

The circulatory system questions

Diagrams—Questions 175–195

175–181. The heart

A. Left atrium
B. Aorta
C. Pulmonary artery
D. Pulmonary veins
E. Inferior vena cava
F. Bicuspid valve
G. Pulmonary valve

175
176
177
178
179
180
181

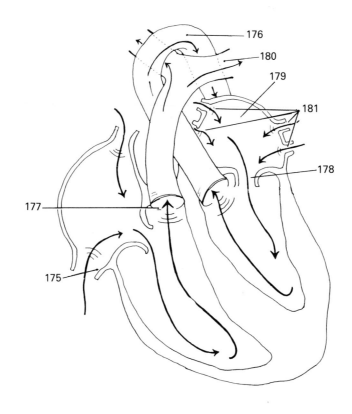

182–188. The arteries

    A. Carotid

    B. Radial

    C. Brachial

    D. Facial

    E. Common iliac

    F. Anterior tibial

    G. Popliteal.

| 182 |
| 183 |
| 184 |
| 185 |
| 186 |
| 187 |
| 188 |

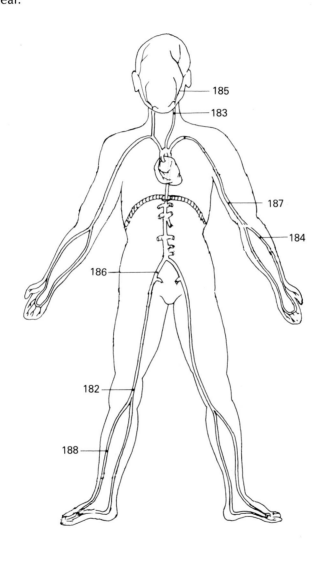

189–195. The veins and lymphatic vessels

A. Jugular vein

B. Axillary nodes

C. Mesenteric nodes

D. Inquinal nodes

E. Thoracic duct

F. Mediastinal nodes

G. Cervical nodes

189

190

191

192

193

194

195

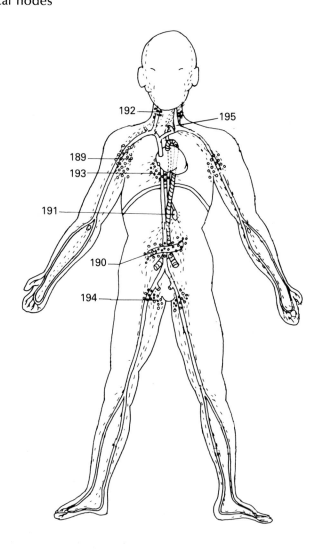

Questions 196–205 are of the multiple choice type

196. **The total volume of blood in the average body is :**   196
    A. 3–4 litres
    B. 5–6 litres
    C. 7–8 litres
    D. 9–10 litres.

197. **The blood is :**   197
    A. slightly acid
    B. slightly alkaline
    C. neutral
    D. strongly alkaline.

198. **Which of the following is the most accurate definition of anaemia?**   198
    A. Bloodlessness
    B. Deficiency of haemoglobin
    C. Deficiency of iron
    D. Deficiency of cyanocobalamin.

199. **Which of the following arteries is not a direct branch of the
    abdominal aorta?**   199
    A. Phrenic
    B. Renal
    C. Internal iliac
    D. Mesenteric.

200. **Which one of the following veins does not enter the inferior vena
    cava?**   200
    A. Gastric
    B. Ovarian
    C. Renal
    D. Phrenic.

201. **Which one of the following statements is true?**   201
    A. Lymphatic capillaries are less permeable than blood capillaries
    B. Lymphatic nodes are similar to glands with ducts
    C. Lymphatic vessels contain numerous valves
    D. The thoracic duct lies entirely within the thorax.

202. **Which one of the following statements is true? Blood travels from:**   202
    A. The left atrium to the aorta
    B. The left ventrical to the vena cava
    C. The right ventricle to the pulmonary artery
    D. The right atrium to the pulmonary veins.

203. **Which one of the following is not a factor which maintains the blood pressure?**

    A. The volume of blood in the blood vessels

    B. The pressure of valves in the veins

    C. The cardiac output

    D. The peripheral resistance.

203

204. **The cardiac cycle normally occurs once in :**

    A. 1 second

    B. 0.1 second

    C. 0.3 second

    D. 0.8 second.

204

205. **Which one of the following will slow the rate of the heart?**

    A. Emotion

    B. Exercise

    C. Physical training

    D. Haemorrhage.

205

Questions 206–254 are of the true/false type.   **T** | **F**

206–209. The heart

    206. lies in front of the oesophagus

    207. lies behind the bronchus

    208. lies with its apex in contact with the diaphragm

    209. lies with its base tilted towards the left.

210–213. The coronary sinus

    210. is a cavity in the skull

    211. is part of the nerve supply to the heart

    212. is to be found in the right atrium

    213. contains venous blood.

214–217. The inferior vena cava

    214. is formed by the junction of the common iliac veins

    215. enters the right atrium

    216. passes through the diaphragm

    217. lies to the left of the aorta.

218–221. Erythrocytes

    218. have a phagocytic action

    219. synthesise haemoglobin

    220. transport oxygen

    221. are greater in number in women than in men.

222–225. The spleen

    222. is essential for life

    223. can produce extra erythrocytes in an emergency

    224. destroys erythrocytes

    225. contains lymphocytes.

226–229. Diastole is part of the cardiac cycle. During diastole :

    226. the atria and ventricles are relaxed

    227. the atrio-ventricular valves are closed

    228. the blood is entering the heart by the pulmonary veins

    229. the blood pressure is increased.

230–234. If a blood transfusion is necessary a person who belongs to group :

    230. O can give blood to group A

    231. AB can receive blood from group A

    232. B can receive blood from group AB

    233. A can give blood to group B.

234–237. A thrombus :   T | F

    234. is a clot formation in a blood vessel

    235. is common in the veins of the leg

    236. is the same as an embolus

    237. can be prevented by heparin.

238–241. The blood pressure :

    238. falls in shock

    239. falls in immobility in the upright position

    240. rises in cold conditions

    241. falls in old age.

242–245. Venous blood returns to the heart by :

    242. contraction of the heart

    243. gravity

    244. the sucking action of the diaphragm

    245. the 'milking' action of the muscles.

246–249. When the skin arterioles constrict :

    246. heat is lost from the body

    247. the blood pressure rises

    248. the pulse rate increases

    249. the skin becomes pale.

250–253. Osmotic pressure is the force which :

    250. draws tissue fluid through the walls of the capillaries into the blood

    251. pushes the fluid from the blood to the tissue cells

    252. returns the blood to the heart

    253. sends blood into the general circulation.

Questions 254–265 are of the matching items type.

254–256. From the list on the left select the tissue which forms each part of the wall of the heart listed on the right.

A. Areolar tissue	254. Endocardium	254
B. Cardiac muscle tissue	255. Myocardium	255
C. Fibrous tissue	256. Pericardium.	256
D. Squamous epithelium		
E. Voluntary muscle tissue		

257–259. From the list on the left select the tissue which forms each part of the wall of the arteries on the right.

A. Areolar tissue	257. Tunica adventitia	257
B. Cardiac muscle tissue	258. Tunica interna	258
C. Elastic fibrous tissue	259. Tunica media.	259
D. Squamous epithelium		
E. Involuntary muscle tissue		

260–262. From the list on the left select the statement which describes the cells on the right.

A. Help in the clotting of blood	260. Erythrocytes	260
B. Contain fibrinogen	261. Leucocytes	261
C. Help in the formation of antibodies	262. Thrombocytes.	262
D. Contain calcium		
E. Contain iron		

263–265. From the list on the left select the substance present in the plasma which is best described by each word on the right.

A. Albumen	263. Mineral	263
B. Enzyme	264. Protein	264
C. Glycerol	265. Waste.	265
D. Potassium		
E. Urea		

5

The respiratory system

Without oxygen there would be no life. Fortunately, there is plenty of oxygen around. The atmosphere is made up of a mixture of gases of which 20% is oxygen. The oxygen is diluted by 79% nitrogen and other inert gases. There is also a minute quantity of carbon dioxide, 0.04% approximately. In a crowded, badly ventilated room the amount of carbon dioxide in the atmosphere is greatly increased.

Table 5.1 *Composition of the atmosphere*

Inspired air		Expired air	
Oxygen	20%	Oxygen	16%
Carbon dioxide	0.04%	Carbon dioxide	4.04%
Nitrogen	78%	Nitrogen	78%
Other inert gases	1%	Other inert gases	1%
Water vapour	variable	Water vapour	saturated

The exchange of oxygen for carbon dioxide is called respiration and it is the function of the respiratory system. Transport from the lungs to the air is by a series of passages. These passages allow the air containing the vital oxygen to enter the lungs and come in close contact with the blood. This part of respiration is called inspiration. Inspiration is followed by expiration and then a pause.

On inspiration, the blood takes up oxygen from the air. On expiration, air containing less oxygen and more carbon dioxide is breathed out. Most of the carbon dioxide has been carried in the blood plasma to the lungs in the form of *carbonic acid* or *sodium bicarbonate*.

The interchange of gases between the air in the lungs and the blood is called *external res-*

piration. Internal respiration is the interchange between the blood in the capillaries and the tissue cells.

The organs of the respiratory system are the air passages and the lungs. The air passages consist of the nose, the pharynx, the larynx, the trachea and the bronchi. The lungs consist of the bronchi, the bronchioles and the air sacs or alveoli. Because the nose and the larynx are parts of the air passages, two related functions of the respiratory system are smell and speech.

THE AIR PASSAGES

The nose

The nose consists of two parts: the external nose and the nasal cavity.

The external nose protrudes from the face and has a skeleton which is composed of cartilage in its lower part. The upper part, or bridge of the nose, consists of the two *nasal bones.*

The nasal cavity is a large cavity in the skull which is divided into two parts by a septum. Projecting from the walls of this cavity are the upper, middle and lower *conchae* (turbinate bones). These are scroll shaped bones under which are the openings into the nasal sinuses. The septum and the conchae greatly increase the surface area of the nasal cavity. This increase in surface area means that there is a corresponding increase in the lining tissue of the nose which consists of ciliated columnar epithelium (mucous membrane), continuous with the mucous membrane lining the sinuses and the nasal part of the pharynx. This membrane has an important function.

As air is breathed in through the nostrils (the anterior nares), it comes in contact with the mucous membrane. The mucus makes the lining moist and sticky, and it is warm because it has a rich blood supply. The air, therefore, is warmed and moistened. As the mucus is sticky, particles of dust, bacteria and other impurities adhere to it. Tiny hairlike processes, or cilia, project from the epithelium and have a lashing movement which moves the mucus in one direction, into the throat where it is

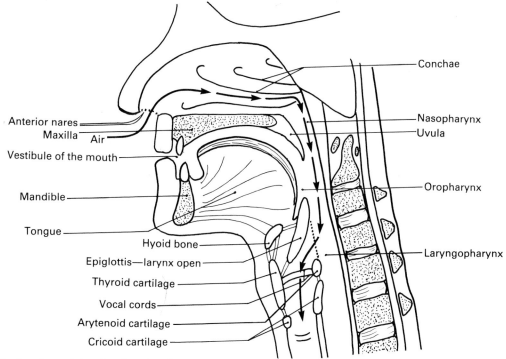

Fig. 5.1 Section through head and neck

Conchae

Nasopharynx
Uvula

Oropharynx

Laryngopharynx

Anterior nares
Maxilla
Air
Vestibule of the mouth

Mandible

Tongue

Hyoid bone
Epiglottis—larynx open
Thyroid cartilage
Vocal cords
Arytenoid cartilage
Cricoid cartilage

swallowed. In this way the lining of the nose acts as a filter for the air.

If you have a cold, the lining of the nose becomes inflamed and secretes more mucus. You become aware of this mucus and call it catarrh. The infection can spread easily from the nose into the throat and sinuses of the skull because of the continuity of the mucous membrane lining the cavities.

The sense of smell

High up in the roof of the nose are the endings of the nerve of smell—the *olfactory nerve*. The nerve endings are present in the mucous membrane, and the nerve fibres enter the skull through the perforated plate of the ethmoid bone. These nerve fibres carry the impulse to the part of the brain which interprets smell. Odours are in the form of gases mixed with air. Some smells, usually the unpleasant ones, are so powerful that they can reach the roof of the nose whilst other weaker smells have to be sniffed up.

The pharynx

The pharynx is the throat. It is a muscular tube about 12 cm long lying in front of the cervical vertebrae and behind the nose, the mouth and the larynx. It is lined with mucous membrane and is described in three parts: the nasopharynx, the oropharynx and the laryngopharynx.

The nasopharynx is continuous with the cavity of the nose. The *auditory tubes* which carry air to the middle ear have openings into the nasopharynx. These tubes are essential for hearing. This part of the pharynx contains some lymphoid tissue called the pharyngeal tonsils. These may be overgrown in young children causing obstruction of the passage for air. The enlarged masses of lymphoid tissue are called *adenoids* and are the reason why some children breathe through the mouth.

The oropharynx is separated from the cavity of the mouth by two folds of mucous membrane (called the *fauces*), hanging down from the soft palate. Between these folds lie the oral tonsils. A muscular projection of the palate lies

in the middle of the arch formed by these folds. This is the *uvula*.

The laryngopharynx is the part which opens into both the larynx and the oesophagus. This makes the oral and laryngeal parts of the pharynx a common passage for food and air. This combined function makes the pharynx resemble the junction of four busy streets. If the traffic lights are not working , the streets may become 'choked' with traffic.

Air passes from the nose down the nasopharynx, the oropharynx and the laryngopharynx into the larynx. Food passes from the mouth through the oropharynx and laryngopharynx into the oesophagus. Once food, mucus and saliva have passed through the fauces into the pharynx, swallowing becomes an involuntary action. If breathing takes place while food is in the pharynx, it will be inhaled into the larynx and cause choking, which we describe as 'food going down the wrong way.' To prevent this happening, the entrance to the nasopharynx constricts and prevents the food from going up into the nose. The *epiglottis* (part of the larynx) closes the inlet to the larynx and food is directed down into the oesophagus.

When choking occurs, coughing will usually dislodge the piece of food. An unconscious patient, however, can neither swallow nor cough, and if food or mucus and saliva enter his air passages, they will be inhaled into the lungs with possible fatal results. The nursing

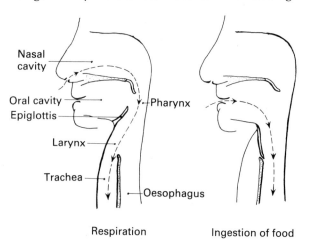

Respiration   Ingestion of food

Fig. 5.2 Diagrammatic section of pharynx

care of such a patient involves keeping the pharynx free of secretions. This is done by using an electric sucker and swabbing the mouth. The patient is fed by a tube which is passed through the nose into the pharynx and then down the oesophagus into the stomach.

When a patient is being prepared for an anaesthetic no food is given for the preceding four hours. This is because the anaesthetic renders the patient unconscious and temporarily paralyses his swallowing and coughing reflexes. Some anaesthetics irritate the stomach causing vomiting. If there is any food in the stomach, it will pass into the pharynx and may enter the larynx and be inhaled into the lungs. The conscious person is continually swallowing mucus and saliva, but when a patient is anaesthetised these substances would trickle down into the lungs. To prevent this happening, drugs such as atropine are given before operation to dry up the secretions.

The larynx

As well as being an air passage the larynx is the voice box. It can be felt at the top of the neck and is made of several cartilages joined by ligaments. The largest of these cartilages is the *thyroid* cartilage. It consists of two plates of hyaline cartilage fused together in front but incomplete at the back, rather like a partly opened book. Below the thyroid cartilage is the *cricoid* cartilage which is shaped like a signet ring. The wide part of the ring lies posteriorly and fits in between the plates of the thyroid cartilage. Situated at the top of the posterior part of the cricoid are two small *arytenoid* cartilages. These cartilages have the vocal cords attached to them. The fourth cartilage is the *epiglottis*. It is a leaf-shaped structure attached to the inner surface of the thyroid cartilage. During swallowing, the larynx rises and the epiglottis covers over the inlet (See Figs. 5.1 and 5.2).

The voice

The larynx is lined with mucous membrane which becomes ciliated in the lower part. In the upper part, two folds of this membrane form the *vocal cords*. These cords stretch across from the thyroid cartilage in front to the arytenoid cartilages at the back, narrowing the air passage. As air from the lungs is forced through the cords the voice is produced. The brain, the tongue, the lips, the facial muscles and the air sinuses all help to convert these sounds into speech.

The vocal cords can be tightened or slackened like a violin string to give pitch to the voice. At puberty a boy's larynx will enlarge with the result that the vocal cords are longer than a girl's. His voice is said to 'break', producing a lower pitch. This larger larynx in a man is sometimes very prominent and is called his 'Adam's apple'.

The loudness of the voice depends on the amount of air which is forced through the cords making them vibrate. The resonance and quality of the voice depend on the hollow air sinuses in the skull, the shape of the mouth and the position of the tongue.

Laryngitis is inflammation of the larynx. The vocal cords become swollen and the voice becomes a whisper. In sinusitis the voice loses its resonance.

The trachea

The trachea is the windpipe. It is continuous with the larynx and is about 10 cm long. It con-

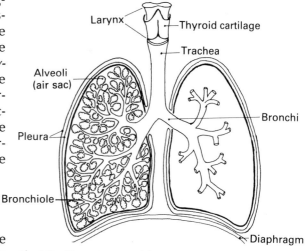

Fig. 5.3 Air passages and lungs

sists of C-shaped cartilages joined by muscle and fibrous tissue. The rings of cartilage can be felt in front of the neck. The back of the trachea is soft and lies anterior to the oesophagus. It is lined with ciliated mucous membrane.

The bronchi

At about the middle of the thorax the trachea divides to form the right and left bronchus. The bronchi enter the lungs, the right one dividing into three and the left one into two branches.

These branches divide again and again getting smaller each time. The bronchi have a similar structure to the trachea except that the rings of cartilage are complete.

If you study Figure 5.3 you will see that the system of air passages looks like an inverted tree. The trachea is the trunk and the bronchi the limbs and branches. The twigs of the bronchial tree are the *bronchioles* which are the smallest of the air passages. The bronchioles lie entirely within the lungs and have no cartilagenous rings. They consist of involuntary muscle tissue and elastic fibrous tissue. From the trachea right down to the smallest bronchiole the lining is ciliated mucous membrane.

The bronchioles end in *alveolar* ducts and *alveoli*. These are thin-walled air sacs consisting of squamous epithelium. They are like balloons and are surrounded by a network of capillaries from the pulmonary circulation. This is where the interchange of gases takes place.

The air is moistened and warmed as it passes down the bronchial tree. The cilia moves the mucus, with any inhaled particles, up out of the lungs into the pharynx where it is swallowed. Irritants which have been inhaled may cause an excess of mucus to be secreted. When it is coughed up, this mucus may be thin and watery or thick and sticky. We call it *sputum* and the act of coughing it up is called expectoration.

The rings of cartilage in the bronchi hold the passages open. The muscular walls of the bronchioles, however, are under nervous control. When they contract the passage becomes narrow and when they relax the passage is dilated. In allergic conditions such as *asthma*, the muscular wall goes into spasm, the mucous lining becomes oedematous, the patient has difficulty in breathing and becomes very distressed. Chronic *bronchitis* and *emphysema* are other common diseases which obstruct the airway. The mucous lining is inflamed and swollen, obstructing the air flow, and the alveoli become distended with air which is trapped in them.

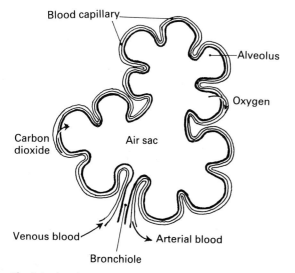

Fig. 5.4 An air sac

THE LUNGS

The lungs are cone-shaped spongy organs situated in the thorax on either side of the heart. As the heart lies slightly over towards the left side, the left lung is smaller then the right one. The base of each lung rests on the diaphragm and the apex extends up into the neck just behind the clavicle.

Each lung consists of lobes and each lobe is made up of lobules. There are three lobes in the right lung and two lobes in the left lung. On the medial side of each lung there is a depression called the hilus. This is where the bronchus, pulmonary artery, bronchial artery and nerves enter the lung and the two pulmonary veins, the bronchial veins and the lymphatic vessels leave. Each lung is made up of all these structures along with the branches of the bronchi, the bronchioles and the alveoli. Elastic connective tissue forms a delicate network holding the various parts together.

The pleura

On the outside of each lung is a serous membrane called the pleura. This membrane is a double sac. The outer (parietal) layer lines the chest wall and covers the upper surface of the diaphragm. The inner (visceral) layer is attached to the surface of the lung and these two layers are always in contact. The pleura secretes a serous fluid which lies between the two layers and prevents them from rubbing on each other during breathing. Inflammation of the pleura is called *pleurisy*. In pleurisy pain is experienced at the end of a deep inspiration when the pleura is stretched and there is friction between the inflamed surfaces.

THE MECHANISM OF RESPIRATION

Respiration is the passage of air in and out of the lungs. This occurs about 16 to 18 times each minute. The amount of air going in and out is called the *tidal volume* and is about 400 ml. During the deepest possible inspiration the amount of air taken in is about 4000 ml and is called the *vital capacity*.

The muscles responsible for respiration are the *diaphragm* and the *intercostal* muscles. The diaphragm forms the dome-shaped floor of the thorax. It flattens out when it contracts, thus increasing the depth of the thorax on inspiration. At the same time the intercostal muscles contract and raise the ribs upwards and outwards. The thorax is increased in size in all directions and air passes in through the air passages. The lungs stretch because of their elasticity and fill up the space created. On expiration, the diaphragm and intercostal muscles relax, pressure is exerted on the elastic lungs, they recoil and air is expelled. There is always about 1500 ml of air left in the lungs at the end of expiration. This is called the *residual volume*.

Other muscles are involved in deep or difficult breathing. These are the abdominal muscles and some of the neck and shoulder girdle muscles. Patients who have undergone abdominal surgery may not cough adequately

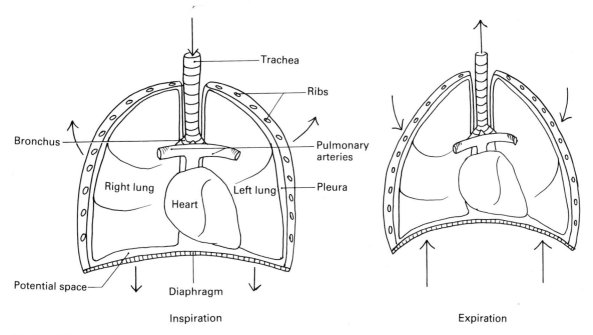

Inspiration

Expiration

Fig. 5.5 Diagrammatic representation of the mechanism of respiration. Diaphragm and lungs

because it hurts the wound and so they risk developing post-operative pneumonia. In this condition, inflammation of the alveoli occurs as a result of failure to clear the mucus from the lungs.

Patients suffering from dyspnoea (difficulty in breathing) should be nursed in the upright position and may be given a bed table to lean on. This allows the patient to fix his shoulder girdle and to use the shoulder muscles to help raise his chest. This makes breathing a little easier.

Breathing is a voluntary action but it is controlled by the brain. If breathing stops for more than three minutes permanent brain damage or even death will result. If you try holding your breath you will find that long before the three minutes are up an involuntary expiration has taken place. There is a special respiration centre in the medulla of the brain (p. 142) which is stimulated by the amount of carbon dioxide in the blood. When the carbon dioxide reaches a certain level involuntary breathing occurs. The amount of CO_2 in the blood also controls the depth of respiration. Increased muscle action produces more carbon dioxide, therefore exercise will increase the rate and the depth of respiration.

When a nurse is recording a patient's respirations she must not only count the rate but she must also notice the depth of respiration and where the movements occur. It is also necessary to observe the patient's colour. An unconscious patient's respiration may be so shallow that the nurse cannot see much chest movement at all. She need not worry very much so long as the patient's colour is good, indicating that he is getting enough oxygen. If, however, his colour is poor in spite of deep inspirations, there is some obstruction of the air passages. His tongue may have fallen back into the pharynx or mucus may be collecting there and blocking the entrance to the larynx. Immediate action must be taken to clear the airway or the patient may die.

Respiratory system questions

Diagrams—Questions 266–278

266–272. The air passages and lungs
- A. Trachea
- B. Right bronchus
- C. Bronchioles
- D. Alevoli
- E. Pleura
- F. Thyroid cartilage
- G. Diaphragm

266
267
268
269
270
271
272

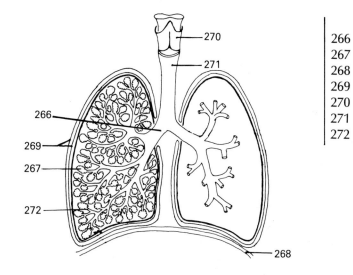

273–278. Section through head and neck
- A. Uvula
- B. Pharynx
- C. Epiglottis
- D. Oesophagus
- E. Larynx
- F. Hyoid bone

273
274
275
276
277
278

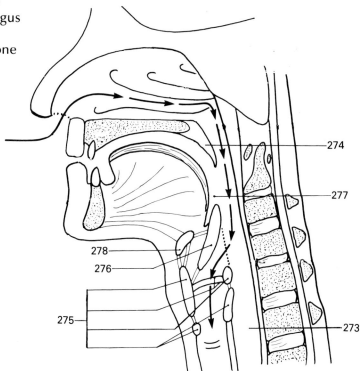

Questions 279–288 are of the multiple choice type

279. **The amount of air entering and leaving the lungs during normal respiration is :**
   A. 200 ml
   B. 400 ml
   C. 2000 ml
   D. 4000 ml.

280. **The percentage of oxygen in inspired air is :**
   A. 16%
   B. 20%
   C. 0.04%
   D. 78%.

281. **The percentage of nitrogen in expired air is :**
   A. 16%
   B. 20%
   C. 60%
   D. 78%.

282. **The conchae are :**
   A. part of the lung
   B. part of the larynx
   C. bones in the nose
   D. the openings into the sinuses.

283. **Which one of the following bones forms the septum of the nose?**
   A. The lacrimal
   B. The maxilla
   C. The nasal
   D. The vomer.

284. **The auditory tubes open into one of the following :**
   A. the nose
   B. the nasopharynx
   C. the oropharynx
   D. the laryngopharynx.

285. **The lining of the nasal sinuses is :**
   A. cuboid epithelium
   B. ciliated epithelium
   C. squamous epithelium
   D. transitional epithelium.

286. **Resonance of the voice depends on the :**
    A. force of air from the lungs
    B. tension in the vocal chords
    C. nasal sinuses
    D. position of the uvula.

287. **The left bronchus :**
    A. lies just above the diaphragm
    B. recoils during expiration
    C. has C-shaped rings of cartilage
    D. divides into two branches.

288. **Atropine is given pre-operatively to :**
    A. act as a sedative
    B. dry up secretions
    C. prevent coughing
    D. prevent vomiting.

286

287

288

Questions 289–320 are of the true/false type   T | F

289–292. The adenoids are :
    289. laryngeal cartilages
    290. lymphoid tissue
    291. oral tonsils
    292. pharyngeal tonsils.

293–296. The vocal cords are attached to the :
    293. thyroid cartilage
    294. cricoid cartilage
    295. arytenoid cartilage
    296. epiglottis.

297–300. The trachea :
    297. is lined with ciliated mucous membrane
    298. is made of involuntary muscle tissue only
    299. joins the larynx to the bronchioles
    300. lies in front of the oesophagus.

301–304. The bronchioles are :
    301. made of cartilage
    302. made of muscle tissue
    303. lined with squamous epithelium
    304. lined with ciliated columnar epithelium.

305–308. The lungs :
    305. are identical in size
    306. have no lymphatic vessels
    307. lie in one pleural cavity
    308. contain a great deal of elastic tissue.

309–312. In the lungs :
    309. mucus is moved upwards by peristalsis
    310. expiration is the result of recoil of the elastic tissue
    311. the parietal layer of the pleura remains in contact with the visceral layer
    312. the pulmonary artery contains oxygenated blood.

313–316. The alveoli :
    313. are made of squamous epithelium
    314. are lined with ciliated columnar epithelium
    315. are surrounded by capillaries from the bronchial artery
    316. recoil during expiration.

317–320. The diaphragm :
    317. has several openings in it
    318. is dome-shaped during inspiration
    319. flattens when it contracts
    320. forms the roof of the abdomen.

Questions 321–326 are of the matching items type.

321–323. From the list on the left select a sign or symptom of each disease on the right.

A. the walls of the bronchi constrict	321. asthma	321
B. the alveoli are distended	322. emphysema	322
C. expiration is difficult and painful	323. pleurisy.	323
D. there is pain on inspiration		
E. the walls of the bronchioles go into spasm		

324–326. From the list on the left select the volume of air involved in the list on the right.

A. 250 ml	324. residual air	324
B. 400 ml	325. tidal air	325
C. 1500 ml	326. vital capacity.	326
D. 4000 ml		
E. 4500 ml		

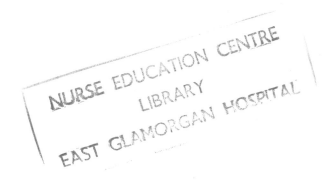

6

The digestive system

The digestive system is a collection of organs which are concerned with all aspects of food. This system takes in food, swallows it, digests it, absorbs it and gets rid of the residue.

FOOD AND ITS USES

Food is essential to the human body. People die of starvation in countries where poverty and ignorance of food values are complace and where famines are not unknown. Even in our own country, lonely old people are often brought into hospital suffering from malnutrition. This is not the same as starvation but is the result of not taking the correct types of food. Tea and buns taken three times a day is rather like filling the petrol tank of a car with water and expecting it to go!

We must have *carbohydrates* and *fats* to provide the fuel to keep going. *Protein, mineral salts* and *vitamins* are necessary to replace and repair worn out parts. *Water* is essential to replace the fluid which is continually being lost and *roughage* is needed to help get rid of the waste.

Carbohydrates

The foods required for energy and heat are called carbohydrate foods because they contain carbon, hydrogen and oxygen. Some of the carbohydrates are very insoluble and require a lot of digesting before they can be absorbed into the blood stream and used as fuel. These are the *starchy* foods, potatoes and all foods made from flour. Sugars, such as cane and beet sugars (*sucrose*), the sugar of milk (*lactose*) and the sugar of malt (*maltose*) are less insoluable and therefore are more easily digested. All the carbohydrate foods, starches and sugars, must be converted into *glucose* by the digestive juices before they can be utilised by the body. However, glucose in powdered form can be taken in food, especially in fruit drinks. It requires no digestion and can be absorbed in the stomach. Glucose is a readily available source of energy and can be given directly into the blood stream by intravenous infusion.

Fats

Fatty foods are rather like the carbohydrates, both in their composition and their action. They provide energy and heat. They also provide food stores, the adipose tissue of the body and protective coverings for some organs. Butter, cream, egg yolks, fish and the fat of meat are fatty foods. Nuts and oils are another source of fat in the diet. Fats are broken down into *fatty acids* and *glycerol* by the bile and pancreatic juices.

Protein

Protein foods contain nitrogen in addition to carbon, hydrogen and oxygen. They are called the nitrogenous foods and are required to build and replace the protoplasm of the body cells. The best type of protein is obtained from animal flesh, meat and fish. Milk, egg white, and cheese and some vegetables, particularly peas, beans and lentils, are also good sources of protein. Protein foods are broken down by the digestive juices into *amino acids* before they can be absorbed and utilised.

Water

Water is absolutely essential for life as it forms nearly one quarter of the body weight. It forms all the body fluids and is necessary for the formation of the secretions of the glands. The amount of water in the body is about 45 litres. 30 litres are present inside the cells and 15 litres lie outside as extracellular fluid which is the tissue fluid and the plasma. If the body is depleted of fluid the signs and symptoms of dehydration appear. These are thirst, dry mouth, slack inelastic skin, sunken eyes and low blood pressure. If untreated, coma and death will result. The amount of fluid taken in each day must be balanced by the output. The importance of maintaining intake and output records for certain patients must be understood by even the most junior nurse.

Mineral salts

An electrolyte is a solution of a substance (a mineral salt) which is capable of conducting electricity. The important mineral salts are *sodium* and *potassium*. Mineral salts are taken in the diet and are excreted by the kidneys, the skin and the bowel. In this way, the electrolyte balance is maintained. This balance is essential as the osmotic pressure of the fluid surrounding the body cells depends on it. If the extracellular fluid contains an excess of mineral salts in solution, the intracellular fluid will be drawn out through the cell wall by osmosis resulting in the cells becoming shrivelled up (see Chapter 1). Sodium and potassium are present in most foods and sodium chloride (table salt) is a common ingredient in cooking. Sodium chloride can be given by intravenous infusion, provided the solution is the same strength as the body fluids. Normal saline contain 0.9 G sodium chloride in 100 ml of water which means that it has the same osmotic pressure as blood.

Other mineral salts are *calcium, phosphorus, iodine* and *iron*. Calcium and phosphorus are required for hardening bone and teeth. Calcium is also necessary for the conducting of impulses along the nerves and for the clotting of blood. Calcium is present in milk, cheese, eggs and green vegetables. Phosphorus is present in most foods. Iodine is essential for the functioning of the thyroid gland and is present in sea foods and green vegetables.

Iron is obtained from vegetables, especially spinach, egg yolk and meat. It is required for the formation of haemoglobin.

Vitamins

Vitamins are chemical substances found in certain foods and they are necessary for perfect health. Their existence was discovered in 1912, since when many of the vitamin deficiency diseases which were prevalent at the beginning of the century have become rare.

Vitamins A, D, E and K are fat soluble. Vitamins B and C are soluble in water and are easily destroyed by cooking.

Vitamin A

Vitamin A is found in all fatty foods, milk, cheese, butter, liver and fish liver oils. It can be made in the body from a substance called *carotene* which is present in brightly coloured vegetables such as carrots, tomatoes and the outer leaves of cabbage and lettuce. This vitamin keeps the mucous membrane and the eyes in a healthy condition by helping to fight infection. It also prevents *night blindness*. If your diet contains an adequate supply of vitamin A, you will find it fairly easy to see where you are when you go into a dark room from a brightly lit one.

Vitamin D

Vitamin D is found in dairy produce and also in fatty fish, salmon, cod, herring and sardines. It can also be built up in the body. The ultra-violet rays from the sun act on a fatty substance in the skin called *ergosterol* which produces vitamin D. For this reason, exposure to the sun's rays is beneficial, especially during the growing period, because calcium cannot be absorbed unless vitamin D is present.

If a child lacks vitamin D he will suffer from *rickets*. In this condition, calcium fails to be laid down in the bones and they become soft and pliable. Young children and pregnant women are given cod liver oil which is an excellent source of both vitamin D and A. However, care must be taken with the dosage as too much can produce toxic symptoms and stones in the kidney.

Vitamin E

Vitamin E is present in egg yolk, milk and green vegetables. It is thought to be necessary for reproduction and for muscle development.

Vitamin K

Vitamin K is found in fish, green vegetables and fruit and is necessary for the clotting of blood.

Vitamin B

There are several closely related vitamins found in the same foods which come under the general heading of vitamin B. These vitamins are found in the husk of wheat, nuts, oatmeal, whole rice, fruit and yeast. They are also present in animal foods such as egg yolk and liver.

This complex vitamin is sometimes called the anti-neuritic vitamin as it is required for a healthy nervous system. Deficiency of vitamin B_1 is common in countries where polished rice is the staple diet. A disease called *beri-beri* is the result and the patients suffer from painful neuritis.

Deficiency of vitamin B_2 causes *stomatitis* (inflammation of the mouth). Vitamin B_2 can be built up by the bacteria in the intestine. Oral antibioties can destroy these bacteria and may result in deficiency of the vitamin.

Vitamin B_{12} is found in animal foods especially liver. It combines with the anti-anaemic factor in the stomach and is carried by the portal vein to the liver for storage. Vitamin B_{12} is required for the normal development of red blood corpuscles in the bone marrow. Its absence is the cause of *pernicious anaemia*.

Vitamin C

Vitamin C is present in citrus fruits, oranges and lemons. It is also present in black currants, rose hips, potatoes, tomatoes and green vegetables. Absence of vitamin C causes scurvy, a condition which used to be common in sailors on long sea voyages. Scurvy is occasionally seen today in old people who have not been feeding themselves properly. The gums become swollen and spongy and there is bleeding into the skin.

Vitamin C is given to young babies in the form of orange juice. It helps in the formation of bones and teeth and is also necessary for the formation of connective tissues. It therefore plays a part in the healing of wounds.

Roughage

Roughage is the indigestible part of food. It is the fibrous part, giving bulk to the food and stimulating bowel action thus preventing constipation.

THE STRUCTURE AND FUNCTION OF THE DIGESTIVE ORGANS

The digestive system is described in two parts: the alimentary canal and the accessory organs.

The *alimentary canal* is a long muscular tube which extends from the mouth to the anus. It is about 9 metres long and acts like a conveyor belt along which the food passes. At various points, the food is mixed with digestive juices. These juices contain *enzymes*. Enzymes are chemical substances which break down complex proteins, carbohydrates and fat into simple soluble substances.

A three-course meal is completely changed in appearance before it is halfway through the canal. The teeth have chopped up large particles into smaller ones. The act of chewing (mastication) mixes these particles with saliva. The resulting soft ball of food is swallowed and passes down the pharynx and oesophagus into the stomach. In the stomach the food is mixed with gastric juice and becomes softened and more fluid. This fluid now passes into the small intestine where it is mixed with pancreatic juice, bile and intestinal juice. All these juices contain enzymes which convert the food into a soluble form. The potatoes and sugar are now *glucose*, the meat is in the form

of *amino acids* and the fat has been converted into *fatty acids* and *glycerol*. These substances are absorbed through the walls of the small intestine into the blood stream, and are ready to be converted into energy as well as to build up body cells. The process of converting food into energy is called *metabolism*.

The food residue, the indigestible parts, are passed on into the large intestine and are eventually excreted as *faeces*.

THE STRUCTURE OF THE ALIMENTARY CANAL

Although the alimentary canal is made up of different organs, their structure is similar.

The muscular coat

The canal is made of involuntary muscle tissue which has circular and longitudinal fibres. When the circular muscles contract the food is pushed along into the next bit of the canal. This movement is called *peristalsis*. If the muscular coat loses its tone, peristalsis ceases and an obstruction occurs. Absorption cannot then take place, vomiting occurs, the patient becomes dehydrated and may collapse.

The peritoneum

The covering of the canal is called the peritoneum. It can be compared with the pleura of the lungs and the pericardium of the heart because it is a double sac of serous membrane. The peritoneum secretes serous fluid which prevents friction as the abdominal organs move on each other. One layer of the peritoneum lines the abdominal cavity and the other layer covers the organs. This second layer holds the organs in place and carries their blood vessels and nerves. It also contains a lot of fat.

The two layers of the peritoneum are in contact with each other but there is a potential space between them which is called the peritoneal cavity.

Peritonitis is inflammation of the peritoneum. This is a serious condition as infection can spread easily from one organ to another.

The mucous membrane

The mucous membrane lining the canal secretes a lubricating mucus and contains the digestive glands. In the small intestine, small projections from the lining allow for absorption of the end-products of digestion. Underneath this mucous membrane is a layer of loose connective tissue which contains the blood vessels, nerves and lymphatic vessels. The nerve supply is from the autonomic nervous systems (see p. 147).

The parts of the alimentary canal are:
the mouth
the pharynx
the oesophagus

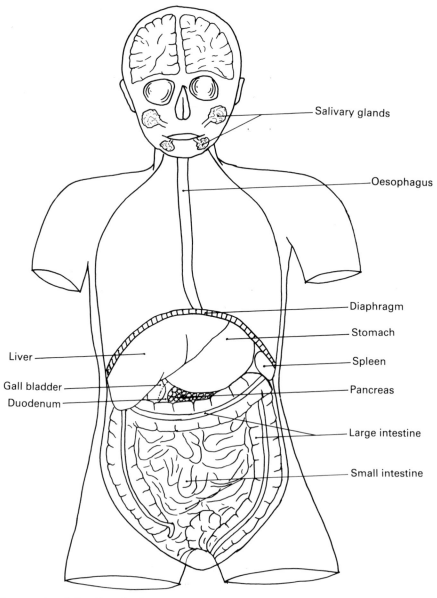

Fig. 6.1 Alimentary canal and digestive glands

the stomach
the small intestine
the large intestine

The accessory organs are:
the salivary glands
the pancreas
the liver

THE MOUTH

The mouth consists of the *vestibule*, which is the part between the lips and the teeth, and the *oral cavity*.

The oral cavity has bony walls with a muscular floor in which the tongue lies. The roof consists of the hard and the soft palates. At the back, the soft palate forms the pillars of the fauces separating the oral cavity from the pharynx. Lining the mouth is mucous membrane which is continuous with the covering of the gums and cheeks.

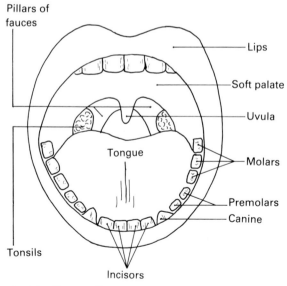

Fig. 6.2 The mouth

The teeth

The teeth perform the important mechanical breakdown of the food. The *incisors* and *canines* are the sharp teeth in front. These teeth bite, cut and tear up the food into little pieces. At the back are the larger flat teeth, the *premolars* and the *molars*, which grind and pulp the food.

The teeth are embedded in sockets in the gums. Every individual has two sets of teeth which are present in the gums at birth. The temporary teeth, of which there are twenty, start to appear when the child is about six months old. They should all be present by the time he is two years old.

There are thirty-two permanent teeth. These teeth start to replace the temporary ones from about the age of six years and are usually all present by the time the child has reached the late teens.

Each tooth has two parts. The crown which is above the gum and the root which is in the tooth socket. The incisors and canines have one root but the other teeth have two and sometimes three roots.

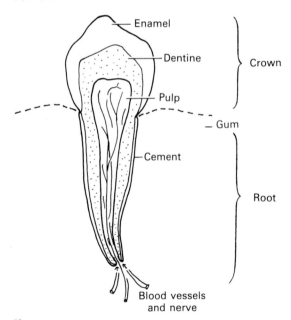

Fig. 6.3 A tooth

The teeth are made of *dentine*, a hard tough yellowish-white tissue. The dentine of the crown is covered by very hard *enamel*. The root is fixed in the socket by a tissue called *cement*. In the centre of each tooth is a cavity, the pulp cavity, which contains blood vessels and nerves.

From infancy onwards, the diet must contain enough calcium, phosphorus and vitamin D to keep the teeth healthy.

The tongue

The tongue is a muscular organ lying in the floor of the mouth; it is attached to the mandible and to a small bone called the hyoid bone. Its surface is covered with a moist pink mucous membrane which is rough in appearance because it is covered with numerous *papillae*. These are small projections which contain microscopic *taste buds*. The taste buds are the endings of the nerve of taste and give the sensations of salt, sweet, sour or bitter of any substance which can be dissolved in water.

The tongue is very mobile and with the cheek muscles it mixes the food with saliva. This is the act of chewing or *mastication* as a result of which a soft ball of food called a *bolus* is formed. It is the beginning of the digestive process. The tongue also plays a part in swallowing, and, of course it is necessary for speech.

The mouth contains many nerve endings in addition to those of taste. We can feel the shape, texture and temperature of anything taken into the mouth. Unpleasant substances are normally rejected immediately. It is as well to remember this when encouraging a patient to take some unpleasant medicine.

Attending to oral hygiene is a very necessary and important nursing duty. The mouth can get dry and sordes or crusts will form from unswallowed particles of food, dried up mucus, saliva and bacteria. This occurs very quickly when a person becomes ill and weak, especially if he is taking very little or no nourishment by mouth. The healthy person's mouth is kept clean by movements of the tongue, eating, drinking and by following proper dental care.

The salivary glands

There are three pairs of salivary glands situated around the mouth. These glands consist of lobules connected together by areolar tis-

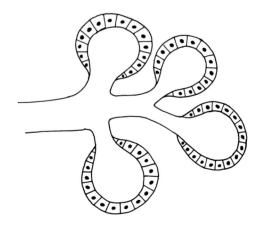

Fig. 6.4 Compound racemose gland

sue. Each lobule has a small duct which joins up with other ducts to form at least one main duct. This type of gland is called a *compound racemose* gland. Each lobule is made up of cells which secrete *saliva.*

Saliva consists of water, mineral salts and an enzyme called ptyalin which starts the digestion of starchy foods. Saliva is slightly acid. It keeps the mouth moist and helps to soften the food. The salivary glands are supplied by the autonomic nervous system and the secretion of saliva is stimulated by the thought, the sight, the smell and the taste of food. This is a very good reason for serving the patient's food punctually.

The salivary glands are in pairs, one on either side of the mouth. They are:
the parotid glands
the submandibular glands
the sublingual glands

The parotid glands are situated just below the ears. Their ducts enter the mouth on the inside of the cheek. *Parotitis* or inflammation of the parotid gland may be due to infection by the virus of mumps or it may be the result of inadequate oral hygiene in a debilitated patient. The infection from the dirty mouth travels along the duct into the gland which becomes swollen and painful.

The submandibular and sublingual glands lie under the mandible and tongue respectively, and pour their secretions into the floor of the mouth.

THE PHARYNX

The pharynx has been described in the preceding chapter (p. 88). The bolus of food formed in the mouth is pushed backwards and upwards against the palate and passes through the fauces into the pharynx. When the bolus or fluid reaches the pharynx, swallowing becomes involuntary. The muscular wall of the pharynx constricts and pushes the food over the epiglottis (which closes the larynx), and on into the oesophagus.

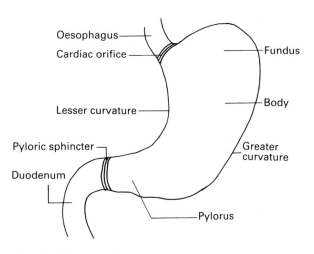

Fig. 6.5 The stomach

THE OESOPHAGUS

The oesophagus is the part of the alimentary canal which lies in the thorax. It extends from the pharynx down behind the heart, through the diaphragm and into the abdomen. It is about 25 cm long and has a covering of elastic fibrous tissue. Liquids and semisolids slide down it assisted by gravity. Solid food is pushed down by *peristalsis*. With each swallow a small quantity of air reaches the stomach. If this air intake is excessive, flatulence will result, and 'wind' is belched up. This may become a very unsociable habit. It is, however, acceptable and necessary for an infant to bring up any swallowed air. This is why a baby should be nursed against his mother's shoulder after being fed.

THE STOMACH

The stomach is a muscular bag which lies under the diaphragm and lower ribs in the left hypochondriac, epigastric and umbilical regions of the abdomen (see p. 11) The oesophagus enters the stomach at the *cardiac orifice*. The part of the stomach above this orifice is the *fundus*. The main part of the stomach is called the *body* and the part which is continuous with the small intestine is the *py-*lorus*. The stomach is often described as a 'J-shaped' organ with a lesser curvature and a greater curvature. The pylorus forms the lower curve of the 'J'.

The stomach is covered on its outside by the peritoneum which attaches it to the posterior abdominal wall. From the greater curvature the peritoneum extends down is front of the abdominal organs like an apron. This is the *greater omentum*. It contains a great deal of fat for which it acts as a storehouse. The omentum also helps to prevent the spread of infection in the abdominal cavity by wrapping itself round the organs.

The muscular wall of the stomach has longitudinal, oblique and circular muscle fibres. Where the pylorus joins the small intestine is a thickened area of circular fibres. This is called the *pyloric sphincter*. A sphincter is a circular muscle which, when it contracts, closes the opening in the centre. The pyloric sphincter controls the amount of food passing into the intestine. Movements of the muscular coat of the stomach churn the food up and mix it with gastric juice.

The mucous membrane lining the stomach contains gastric glands. These are simple tubular glands which pour gastric juice into the stomach. Gastric juice contains water, hydrochloric acid, mineral salts and enzymes as well as the intrinsic factor.

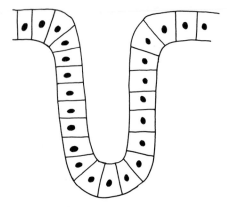

Fig. 6.6 Simple tubular gland

The bolus, when churned up with gastric juice and mucus, becomes more fluid and is called *chyme*. This chyme is acid because of the *hydrochloric acid* content in the gastric juice. The acid helps digestion and kills any bacteria which may have been swallowed with the food.

The enzymes are *pepsin* (which starts the digestion of protein), and *rennin* (which is present in an infant's stomach and curdles the milk). The *intrinsic factor*, or anti-anaemic factor, is also present and is essential for the absorption of vitamin B_{12}.

A normal mixed meal will remain in the stomach for two to four hours but every few minutes a small amount of the food reaches the pyloric sphincter and passes into the small intestine.

If the stomach is irritated by swallowing some obnoxious substance, for example infected food or excess alcohol, the cardiac orifice relaxes and the abdominal wall contracts. The contents are forcibly ejected up the oesophagus into the pharynx. The partly digested food enters the mouth and is expelled. *Vomiting* can also result from some irritation of the area of the brain which contains the vomiting centre. Sea sickness is an example of this type of vomiting.

Gastritis is inflammation of the mucous membrane of the stomach resulting from the ingestion of some irritating substance. It is usually accompanied by nausea and vomiting. *Peptic ulcer* is an ulcer occurring in the mu-cous membrane of those sections of the alimentary tract where gastric juice is present. Some gastric juice enters the first part of the small intestine (the duodenum) when the chyme goes through the pyloric sphincter. If a peptic ulcer occurs in the stomach it is called a gastric ulcer. If it occurs in the duodenum it is called a duodenal ulcer.

THE SMALL INTESTINE

The small intestine or bowel is about six to seven metres in length. It commences at the pyloric sphincter and ends in the right iliac region where it joins the large intestine. It is de-

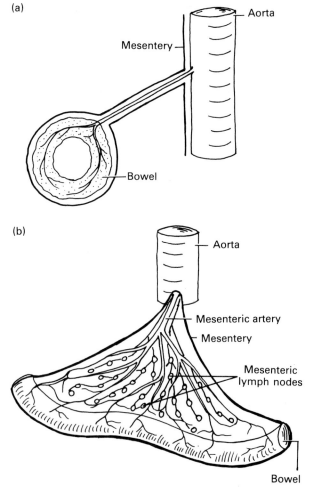

Fig. 6.7 The mesentery

scribed as being in three different parts. The first 25 centimetres is 'C-shaped' and is called the *duodenum*. It surrounds the head of the pancreas. The next two-fifths is called the *jejunum* and the last three-fifths is the *ileum*. This division is only made for descriptive convenience as the small intestine is a continuous tube.

The fold of peritoneum covering the coils of the small intestine is called the *mesentery*. It is fan-shaped (see Fig. 6.7) and attaches the bowel to the posterior abdominal wall. The mesentery contains blood vessels, nerves and lymphatic vessels and nodes.

The mucous membrane of the small intestine is arranged in folds which greatly increase the surface area. It contains intestinal glands. These are simple tubular glands which secrete intestinal juice. Intestinal juice contains several enzymes, namely maltase, sucrase and lactase which complete the digestion of carbohydrates into glucose. Peptidases (erepsin) are also present and they complete the breakdown of protein into amino acids.

Halfway along the duodenum is a small projection or *ampulla* which is where the bile duct joins the pancreatic duct. Where the ampulla opens into the bowel there is a sphincter muscle called the *sphincter* of *Oddi* (See Fig. 6.10).

Pancreatic juice is an alkaline fluid containing enzymes. The enzymes are trypsin, amylase and lipase which act on protein, carbohydrate and fat respectively. Bile is also alkaline and is a yellow-green bitter fluid secreted by the liver and stored in the gall bladder. The function of bile is to emulsify fat. The pancreatic juice and the bile enter the duodenum through the sphincter of Oddi.

The acid chyme in the stomach becomes alkaline chyme in the duodenum. It is moved along by peristalsis and mixed with pancreatic and intestinal juices until digestion is completed. The end products are absorbed through the walls of the *villi* and the residue continues on into the large intestine (Table 6.1).

The villi are tiny finger-like projections which project from the lining of the small intestine. Inside each villus is a network of

Table 6.1 *Food: ingestion, digestion, absorption*

Organ	Movement	Glands	Juices	Enzyme	Acts on	Result
Mouth	Mastication	Salivary Parotid Sub-mandidular Sublingual	Saliva (slightly acid)	Pytalin	Starch	Bolus
Pharynx	Swallowing	—	—	—	—	—
Oesophagus	Peristalsis	—	—	—	—	—
Stomach	Churning	Gastric	Gastric (strongly acid)	Pepsin	Protein	Chyme
Duodenum	Peristalsis	Liver	Bile (alkaline)	—	Fat	Chyme Fat emulsified
—	—	Pancreas	Pancreatic (alkaline)	Amylase Lipase	Starch Fat	Chyme Fat digested → fatty acids & glycerol
Small Intestine	Peristalsis	Intestinal	Intestinal (alkaline)	Sucrase Maltase Lactase Pepsidase (Erepsin)	Cane sugar Malt sugar Milk sugar Protein	Glucose Amino acids
Large intestine	Peristalsis	—	—	—	Water absorbed from residue mixed with bacteria	Faeces

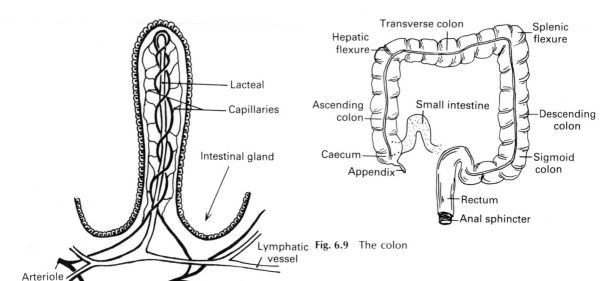

Fig. 6.8 A villus

Fig. 6.9 The colon

blood capillaries and a lymphatic capillary. The glucose and amino acids pass into the blood and the fatty acids and glycerol pass into the lymph. The lymphatic capillary is called a *lacteal* because the fat makes the lymph milky in appearance.

THE LARGE INTESTINE

The large intestine or colon is about 1.5 metres in length. The first part is called the *caecum*. This is a dilated portion, rather like a small pouch, which lies in the right iliac region of the abdomen. The food residue enters the caecum from the ileum through the *ileo-caecal valve*. Leading from the caecum is the worm-like *appendix*. This is a tube, usually about 9 to 10 cm long, which is continuous with the caecum. It has no known function in man but it is a common site for inflammation (appendicitis). A possible cause of appendicitis is irritation by foreign bodies or hard faeces.

Look at Figure 6.9 and you will see that the caecum becomes the *ascending colon*, which bends at the liver (hepatic flexure) and becomes the *transverse colon*. This part crosses

to the right side, bends at the spleen (splenic flexure) and descends to the pelvis. The *descending colon* enters the pelvis where it becomes the *pelvic* or *sigmoid* colon. The pelvic colon forms an 'S'-bend, passing backwards and downwards to become the *rectum*. The rectum ends at the anal canal and the anal sphincters.

The colon is not smooth on the outside like the small intestine. There are three bands of longitudinal muscle fibres which are shorter than the bowel, giving it a puckered appearance.

Because of the shape of the colon a patient receiving an enema must be placed in the left lateral position if at all possible. Fluid entering the rectum when the patient is on his right side would simply run out again.

When the residue of the food reaches the large intestine it is in fluid form. The function of the colon is to remove some of the water and salts by absorption and to convert the waste material into *faeces*. Faeces are normally brown in colour, have a paste-like consistency and contain millions of bacteria. These bacteria multiply rapidly in the intestine and are known to produce some of the B vitamins. They are collectively known as the coliform bacilli and are harmless in the bowel. They are present in large numbers in the faeces and if they should enter any of the other pelvic organs they will cause inflammation. When cleansing a female patient after a bowel movement, care must, therefore, be taken to take the toilet tissue from the front to the back to prevent the spread of bacteria into the vagina.

Defaecation

When the faeces reach the rectum the walls of this organ are stretched and nerves convey a feeling of fullness to the brain. Defaecation is the passing of faeces through the anal canal. The anal canal is about 4 cm long. It has two sphincter muscles: the internal one is controlled by the autonomic nervous system and the external sphincter is under voluntary control. The sphincters relax and the faecal matter is pushed out by the contraction of the walls of the rectum aided by the contraction of the anterior abdominal wall muscles.

Constipation is the condition when there is infrequent defaecation and hard stools which are difficult to pass build up in the rectum. It may occur as a result of the desire to defaecate being suppressed. This suppression by bedridden patients is understandable when you consider the discomfort of using a bedpan. Patients should be allowed to get up to use a commode whenever possible. Other causes of constipation are insufficient roughage in the diet and sluggish bowel movements. The faeces collect in the rectum, more water is absorbed and they become hard and dry and difficult to pass. Constipation should be treated by improving the diet, increasing the fluid intake, taking plenty of exercise and developing a regular bowel habit.

Sometimes it may be necessary to resort to drugs to correct constipation. These drugs are called *purgatives*, *laxatives* or *aperients*. Some of these drugs act by increasing peristalsis, others act by drawing water back out of the walls of the colon to make the faeces more fluid. Other aperients act as lubricants.

Diarrhoea is the passage of frequent loose stools as a result of some irritation such as food poisoning. Insufficient water is absorbed by the colon and the patient may become dehydrated. Inflammation of the colon is called *colitis*. *Enteritis* is inflammation of the small intestine.

THE PANCREAS

The pancreas is a greyish pink gland which is shaped like a fish. The head lies in the curve of the duodenum, the body lies behind the stomach and the tail is in contact with the spleen. The pancreas is a compound gland made up of lobules. Each lobule has a small duct which unites with the others to form a longer duct. The lobules secrete pancreatic juice which is passed into the duodenum through a large duct called the pancreatic duct at the sphincter of Oddi (see Fig. 6.10). Pancreatic juice consists of water, mineral salts and the enzymes trypsin, amylase and lipase.

Scattered throughout this gland are small areas of a different type of tissue. These areas are called the *islets* of *Langerhans* and they produce *insulin*. The islets are endocrine glands and the insulin passes straight into the blood stream. Insulin is necessary for the storage of glucose in the liver and muscles. If it is absent the individual has diabetes. In this case, glucose passes from the blood into the kidneys and is excreted in the urine.

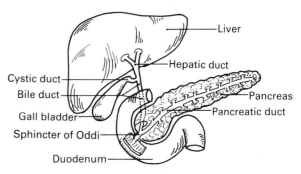

Fig. 6.10 Duodenum, pancreas and liver

THE LIVER

The liver is the largest gland in the body. It lies in the right hypochondriac and epigastric regions of the abdomen. It is wedge-shaped, soft and reddish brown in colour. It is covered by a fold of the peritoneum which attaches it to the diaphragm.

The liver has two lobes. A large right lobe and a smaller left one. The lobes are made up of tiny lobules. Entering the liver on its under surface are the hepatic artery, nerves and the portal vein. Leaving the liver are the bile ducts, the hepatic vein and the lymphatic vessels. The *portal vein* carries blood from the intestines, the stomach and the spleen directly to the liver. This blood contains nutrients from the intestines, bile pigments and iron from the spleen and the anti-anaemic factor which is formed in the stomach.

The liver is the most complex organ in the body. It resembles a large chemical factory receiving its raw materials from the portal vein. It is so active that it generates a great deal of heat. The liver has many functions:

1. Glucose is stored in the form of glycogen which is insoluble. It is turned into glycogen by the action of insulin from the pancreas. If extra glucose is required by the body to cope with an emergency, adrenaline from the adrenal glands turns the glycogen back into glucose.
2. The excess amino acids not required for body building are broken down into glucose and urea. The glucose is used as a fuel and the urea is excreted by the kidneys.
3. It converts the fat which is stored in the body into a form suitable for combustion.
4. It stores iron and vitamins A, B_{12}, D, E and K.
5. It forms vitamin A from carotene.
6. It forms plasma proteins which include the clotting substances.
7. It helps form antibodies.
8. It removes poisons from the blood such as alcohol and toxins resulting from bacterial infection.
9. The liver manufactures bile.

Bile

Bile is a yellowish-green fluid consisting of water, salts, mucus, bile pigments, bile salts and cholesterol. It passes out of the liver through two ducts, one from each lobe. These ducts join to form the hepatic duct which in turn is joined by the cystic duct from the gall bladder. At this junction, the common bile duct is formed. This duct joins the pancreatic duct at the ampulla and opens into the duodenum at the sphincter of Oddi (see Fig. 6.10).

The gall bladder

The gall bladder is a pear-shaped organ lying on the posterior surface of the liver. It acts as a reservoir for the bile which it concentrates by removing some of the water. The wall of the gall bladder is muscular. When a fatty meal has been eaten it contracts and pushes bile down into the duodenum.

The bile emulsifies the fat and helps in its digestion. The bile pigments pass on into the colon, give the faeces their brown colour and act as a deodorant.

If the bile duct becomes blocked by gall stones or infection, *jaundice* will develop. The bile then leaves the liver by the hepatic vein and enters the systemic circulation. It colours the skin and other tissues yellow and is excreted by the kidneys. The urine becomes dark orange in colour. Bile pigments do not reach the colon so the faeces are pale grey in colour, contain undigested fat and are foul smelling.

METABOLISM

Metabolism is the term used to describe the complex process which converts foods into heat and energy. All the body cells require energy for the growth and repair of tissues. Energy is also required for muscle contraction and for the synthesis of secretions by the various glands. All this is under the control of the *thyroid gland* (see p. 169). If this gland is overactive the rate at which the body uses food is increased. Patients suffering from overactivity of the thyroid gland will undergo a test to estimate the basal metabolic rate. This is the rate at which metabolism takes place when the individual has fasted and is at complete rest. The rate is calculated by measuring the amounts of oxygen taken in and of carbon dioxide given out over a given period of time.

The amount of food required in 24 hours varies with age, sex, height and occupation. Carbohydrates, proteins and fatty foods can all be used as fuel, releasing energy and heat. The amount of energy each food substance gives is measured in kilojoules (kj) and the amount of heat given off is measured in kilocalories (kcal). A kilocalorie is equal to a large calorie which is the amount of heat required to raise 1 kg of water through 1° C.

Carbohydrate metabolism

Carbohydrate is the main source of energy in the diet. The glucose is absorbed in the small intestine and carried to the liver by the portal vein. The glucose required for immediate use goes straight through the liver into the blood stream. The rest is stored as glycogen in the liver and muscles. The glycogen in the muscles is converted into glucose which combines with oxygen. This chemical reaction releases the energy which is required for muscle contraction. Heat is produced and the waste products of carbon dioxide and water are formed. Insulin is necessary to convert the glucose to glycogen. Adrenaline and other hormones convert the glycogen back to glucose. Carbohydrates taken in excess of the body's requirement are converted into fat and stored in the adipose tissue.

One gram of carbohydrate provides 17 kilojoules or 4 kilocalories.

Fat metabolism

Fat is absorbed through the walls of the villi into the lacteals and travels up the thoracic duct into the blood stream. The fat is stored in the adipose tissue and can be used for energy when required. Before this can happen the fat must be transported to the liver where it is converted into a form which can be oxidised.

Fat is metabolised with glucose and forms the waste products carbon dioxide and water. However, if glucose is not present in the muscles and fat alone is being used for energy production, poisonous waste products are formed. These waste products are called ketone bodies and their presence in excess in the blood is called ketosis.

Ketosis occurs in *starvation* when there is insufficient carbohydrate in the diet and the body fat is being utilised for energy. It also arises in *diabetes mellitus*. In this condition, the pancreas fails to secrete insulin and glucose is not converted into glycogen. Glucose and acetone will be present in excess in the blood and will be excreted in the urine. Acetone is a ketone body. If a diabetic patient is left untreated he will be poisoned by the accumulation of ketones in the blood and will go into a coma and may die.

One gram of fat provides 38 kilojoules or 9 kilocalories. It therefore produces more than twice the energy and heat provided by carbohydrates.

Protein metabolism

Protein foods are needed for the growth and repair of tissues. The protoplasm of cells is a protein and most of our protein foods consist of animal flesh.

Amino acids are absorbed into the blood stream and are carried by the portal vein to the liver. The amino acids required for growth and repair pass out into the systemic circulation whilst those not required by the tissues return to the liver. The carbon, hydrogen and oxygen part of the protein is separated from the nitrogenous part and is used to provide energy or is stored as fat. The nitrogenous part is excreted by the kidneys in the form of urea.

Amino acids are also formed from the body's own protein. Destruction of body cells goes on all the time and this produces amino acids for growth of new cells. In destructive diseases, such as tuberculosis, high protein diets are given in order to balance the rate of destruction with the rate of repair.

When protein is used for heat and energy it provides the same amount as carbohydrate. One gram of protein provides 17 kilojoules or 4 kilocalories (see Table 6.2).

Table 6.2 *Metabolism*

Food	End product of digestion	Absorbed	Route	Liver	Action	Waste	Excreted by
Carbodydrate	Glucose	Through walls of villi in small intestine into blood capillaries	Portal vein to liver	Stored as glycogen (insulin required)	Carried to muscles— combustion with O_2 releases heat and energy	Carbon dioxide and water	Lungs Skin Kidney Bowel
Protein	Amino acids	Through walls of villi in small intestine into blood capillaries	Portal veins to liver	Excess broken down into— urea and glycogen	Carried to all tissues for growth and repair. Glycogen used for heat and energy	Urea Carbon dioxide and water	Kidneys Lungs Skin Kidney Bowel
Fat	Fatty acids and glycerol	Through walls of villi in small intestine into lymphatic capillaries (lacteals)	Lymphatic system Blood steam Adipose tissue	Prepared for combustion	Combustion in muscles with glucose heat and energy If no glucose (Diabetic)	Carbon dioxide and water Acetone	Lungs Skin Kidney Bowel Kidney

Digestive system questions

Diagrams—Questions 327–351

327–333. Alimentary canal

    A. Oesophagus   327
    B. Stomach   328
    C. Ascending colon   329
    D. Duodenum   330
    E. Caecum   331
    F. Appendix   332
    G. Pelvic colon   333

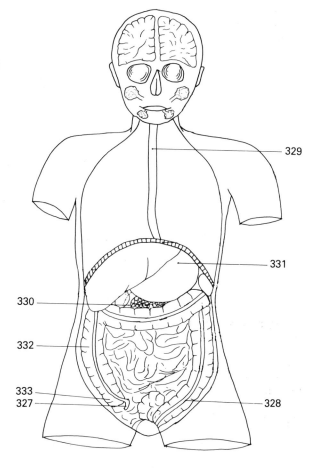

334–340. Mouth and teeth

    A. Fauces   334
    B. Oropharynx   335
    C. Uvula   336
    D. Palate   337
    E. Premolars   338
    F. Canine   339
    G. Incisors   340

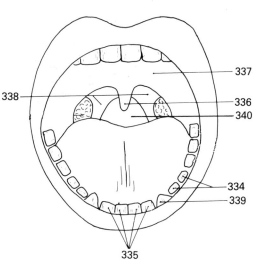

341–345. Stomach

A. Greater curvature   341
B. Fundus   342
C. Pylorus   343
D. Cardiac orifice   344
E. Pyloric sphincter   345

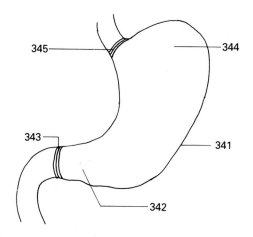

346–351. The liver, pancreas and duodenum

A. Cystic duct   346
B. Sphincter of Oddi   347
C. Right hepatic duct   348
D. Bile duct   349
E. Pancreatic duct   350
F. Gall bladder   351

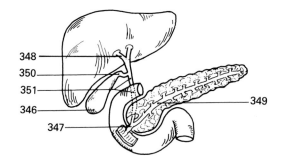

Questions 352–361 are of the multiple choice type.

352. **Which one of the following is a source of protein in the diet?**
    A. Cabbage
    B. Celery
    C. Peas
    D. Tomatoes.

352

353. **Which one of the following is a source of fat in the diet?**
    A. Cane sugar
    B. Egg white
    C. Nuts
    D. White bread.

353

354. **Which one of the following carbohydrates is least easily digested?**
    A. Lactose
    B. Maltose
    C. Sucrose
    D. Starch.

354

355. **The amount of water in the cells of the body is approximately :**
    A. 45 litres
    B. 30 litres
    C. 15 litres
    D. 5 litres.

355

356. **Which one of the following organs is not a part of the digestive system?**
    A. Liver
    B. Oesophagus
    C. Pharynx
    D. Spleen.

356

357. **In the human mouth there are :**
    A. 36 permanent teeth
    B. 20 temporary teeth
    C. 4 incisors
    D. 8 canines.

357

358. **The tongue :**
    A. is attached to the maxilla
    B. is attached to the hyoid bone
    C. is covered with ciliated mucous membrane
    D. contains many taste buds on its inferior surface.

358

359. **Which one of the following is not a salivary gland?**
   A. Parotid
   B. Pineal
   C. Submandibular
   D. Sublingual.

360. **The oesophagus :**
   A. is approximately 30 cm long
   B. lies in front of the trachea
   C. lies behind the aorta
   D. passes through the diaphragm.

361. **To which one of the following parts of the intestine is the appendix attached?**
   A. Caecum
   B. Duodenum
   C. Ileum
   D. Sigmoid colon.

Questions 362–401 are of the true/false type.

362–365. Of the essential food substances :
362. carbohydrate provides energy
363. fats transport vitamins C and B
364. minerals are necessary for fluid balance
365. protein is necessary for the formation of blood.

366–369. Protein :
366. can be used for heat and energy
367. can be changed into urea in the kidneys
368. is absorbed in the form of amino acids
369. is necessary for the growth of tissue.

370–373. Glucose :
370. can be stored unaltered in the liver
371. if taken in excess can be stored as fat
372. is the end product of the digestion of carbohydrate
373. helps to maintain the body temperature.

374–377. The stomach :
374. is covered by the greater omentum
375. joins the duodenum at the pyloric sphincter
376. lies in the left lumbar region of the abdomen
377. lies behind the pancreas.

378–381. The mesentery :
378. contains digestive glands
379. contains lymphatic glands
380. covers the ileum
381. is part of the peritoneum.

382–385. The portal vein carries :
382. bile to the liver
383. glucose to the liver
384. fat to the liver
385. iron to the liver.

386–389. Bile is :
386. a digestive enzyme
387. an emulsifying agent
388. present in the faeces of a jaundiced patient
389. secreted by the gall bladder.

390–393. Urea is :

     390. a mineral salt

     391. the waste product of protein metabolism

     392. formed in the liver

     393. excreted in the faeces.

394–397. Metabolism is :

     394. the process of digestion

     395. the production of energy from food

     396. the elimination of waste

     397. controlled by the thyroid gland.

398–401. The villi :

     398. contain blood vessels but no lymphatic vessels

     399. are only present in the jejunum

     400. absorb the end products of digestion

     401. attaches the bowel to the abdominal wall.

T   F

Questions 402–416 are of the matching items type.

402–404. From the list on the left select the statement which describes each substance on the right.

A. Is an enzyme	402. Antianaemic factor	402
B. Is the chemical name for vitamin E	403. Carotine	403
C. Is present in outer leaves of cabbage	404. Ergosterol.	404
D. Is a fatty substance in the skin		
E. Is secreted by the walls of the stomach		

405–407. From the list on the left pair the organs with the functions on the right.

A. Stomach	405. Absorption	405
B. Small intestine	406. Elimination	406
C. Colon	407. Ingestion.	407
D. Oesophagus		
E. Mouth		

408–410. From the list on the left select a function for each organ listed on the right.

A. Secretes bile	408. Pancreas	408
B. Secretes amylase	409. Small intestine	409
C. Secretes maltose	410. Stomach.	410
D. Secretes sucrase		
E. Secretes pepsin		

411–413. From the list on the left select the statement which describes each substance on the right.

A. Is acid in the stomach	411. Bolus	411
B. Is coloured by bile	412. Chyme	412
C. Is a digestive enzyme	413. Faeces.	413
D. Is masticated food		
E. Is a secretion of the pancreas		

414–416. From the list on the left select the statement which describes each word on the right.

A. Is milk sugar.	414. Lacteal	414
B. Is a lymphatic vessel	415. Lactose	415
C. Is part of the stomach	416. Lactase.	416
D. Is a carbohydrate enzyme		
E. Is part of the liver		

7

The skin

The skin is not only a complete covering for the body but it is the largest and one of the most active organs. It has many functions. Under normal circumstances the skin keeps out micro-organisms, is waterproof, excretes waste products, regulates temperature and is an important sensory organ. It deserves to be well cared for and can only function properly if it is kept clean and if air can circulate round it freely. It is, therefore, important that when covered it should be with the correct type of clothing.

Care of the patient's skin, hair and nails is a fundamental part of a nurse's work and observations of any alterations in appearance must be noted. One of the first signs of ill health is hair which has lost its shine. Rashes appear on the skin in infectious diseases and other systemic conditions.

An uncared for skin may be infected by micro-organisms, producing pustules and boils, or it may become infested by animal parasites. The skin can be oily or dry, tight when there is excess fluid in the tissues and loose when there is dehydration. These are only some of the observations a nurse must make of the patient's skin.

Dermatitis means inflammation of the skin. It may occur as a reaction to certain parts of clothing, buckles and watch straps, or to food, animals, plants, drugs, soaps and detergents. Such allergic reactions can be very disabling and may come to dominate the individual's lifestyle.

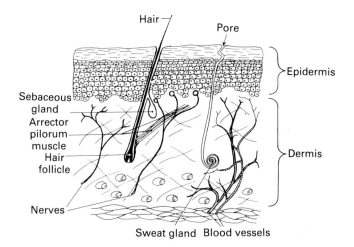

Fig. 7.1 The skin

The skin consists of an outer layer of stratified squamous epithelium called the epidermis and an inner layer of elastic fibrous tissue called the dermis.

THE EPIDERMIS—PROTECTION

The epidermis has a protective function. It acts as a barrier to invading micro-organisms. Once the barrier is broken by injury micro-organisms can enter the underlying tissues and multiply.

Fish and reptiles have obviously scaly skins, like coats of armour, which prevent damage to underlying structures. The human skin appears soft and smooth but under the microscope it can be seen to consist of layers of cells. The upper layers of cells are dead, the protoplasm having been replaced by a horny substance called *keratin.*

The epidermis is thicker is some areas than in others. The thickest areas are the palms of the hands and the soles of the feet. The skin of the eyelids and lips is extremely thin. If the epidermis is subjected to intermittent pressure and friction the hard scaly layers will thicken and form callosities. These areas occur most commonly on the soles of the feet, and on the palms of the hands of people, such as manual workers, who repeatedly use tools which cause pressure and friction.

The dead cells of the epidermis are continually being shed and they are washed off or become detached when clothes are removed each night. Like all dead matter these cells decompose and this is one of the reasons for the unpleasant smell of an unwashed person who sleeps in his clothes. The discarded cells are replaced by others from the lower layers of the epidermis.

The deep layers of the epidermis are the *germinative* layers. They produce the new cells which eventually become the upper layers. Also in these deeper layers is the pigment *melanin.* The colour of the hair and skin depends on the amount of melanin and other pigments present in the epidermis. Exposure to the sun's rays increases the amount of pigment in the epidermis and this in turn protects the deeper layers of the skin from damage by the sun. The ultraviolet rays of the sun manufacture vitamin D by acting on the *erogosterol* in the germinative layer of the skin.

The epidermis is attached to the dermis by projections of the dermis called *papillae.* These papillae appear on the surface as markings. On the finger tips these patterns are the *finger prints* which are different in every individual and are, therefore, so useful for purposes of identification.

If the epidermis is burned or damaged it can repair itself. This does not occur, however, in the dermis. A deep burn involving the whole skin requires a skin graft before it will heal.

THE DERMIS

The dermis consists of white fibrous tissue with many elastic fibres. The elasticity is the reason why the skin fits the body so well. In old age these fibres become less elastic and wrinkles and folds appear in the skin. Under the dermis is a layer of adipose tissue which acts as a food store and also helps to keep the body warm.

In the dermis is a vast network of blood and lymphatic capillaries and nerve endings. These do not enter the epidermis (see Fig. 7.1). Also in the dermis are *sweat glands, hair follicles, sebaceous glands* and small muscles. The blood vessels nourish all these structures, the cells of the dermis, and the deep layer cells of the epidermis.

Unrelieved pressure, such as that caused by lying or sitting in the same position for long periods, occludes the capillaries and causes death of the cells of the dermis. This is commonly the beginning of a pressure sore and it may be present even if the epidermis looks healthy. There will also be pressure on the nerves. Therefore, any complaint of pain should be regarded as a warning symptom.

SENSATION

The skin is the chief, agent of communication between the outside environment and the body. It contains numerous nerve endings which convey the sensations of *touch, temperature, pressure* and *pain* to the brain. It helps protect the body from dangers in the environment.

If these impulses are blocked by injury to the spinal cord they will not reach the brain and the individual will be deprived of skin sensation. This is the problem met with in nursing a paraplegic patient. It would be very easy to burn this patient with a hot water bottle as he would not feel the heat. He feels neither pressure nor pain and, unless turned, would lie quite comfortably in one position until a pressure sore developed. On the other hand, this protective function is greatly increased when one of the other sense organs is missing. Watch a blind person 'seeing' with his hands. The sensation in his skin, especially the tips of the fingers where the nerve endings are most numerous, is most important to him.

EXCRETION

The skin is an excretory organ. Lying in the dermis are *sweat glands*. These are coiled tubular glands with ducts which open on to the surface of the epidermis at pores. *Sweat* is a watery fluid containing electrolytes and some waste substances. It is continually being excreted and evaporated into the surrounding air. This is called insensible sweat as we are unaware of it. It is only when excess is produced that we are conscious of sweating. If exercise is taken in very hot surroundings the sweat glands become very active. Excess water and salt is lost and the individual may become thirsty. Sometimes it is necessary to add extra salt to the diet in order to prevent painful muscle cramps. The cramp is due to the loss of electrolytes.

THE REGULATION OF BODY TEMPERATURE

The skin acts as a thermostat keeping the temperature of the body between 36° and 37°C. Various factors produce heat, muscle contraction being the most important. The digestive organs, particularly the liver, contribute to heat production because of the chemical activities which go on in these organs. Heat is lost from the body in urine, faeces and expired air, but mostly by sweating.

When you get hot the arterioles in the dermis dilate, bringing more blood into the skin capillaries. The skin gets red and hot and heat is lost by radiation and conduction. At the same time, the sweat glands produce more sweat to be evaporated. Evaporation is the turning of a liquid into a gas. This change requires heat which is taken from the skin. There must also be air circulating before evaporation can take place. This is the reason why good ventilation and sensible clothing are important. The more rapid the current of air the quicker the evaporation and the greater the heat loss (as you will soon discover if you sit in a draught).

In cold conditions, when the air temperature is lower than the body temperature, the arterioles in the dermis constrict. Less blood is circulating through the skin, which is white and cold, and less heat is lost to the cold air. The sweat glands produce less sweat and the individual may shiver. Shivering is muscle contraction and occurs in an attempt to balance the heat loss when there is danger of the body temperature falling below normal.

The temperature of the body is controlled by a temperature regulating centre in the brain which is sensitive to the heat of the blood flowing through it. In febrile conditions this centre is upset and if the body temperature rises above 39°C some attempt must be made to lower it. This may be done by tepid sponging. Tepid water is sponged on to the hot skin and allowed to evaporate. This uses up the extra heat and should lower the temperature. In more severe cases, the patient may be covered by a wet sheet and an electric fan used to speed up the rate of evaporation.

HAIR AND NAILS

Hair and nails are derived from the same tissue as the epidermis.

Nails are the equivalent of the claws of animals and birds. In the human, nails protect the very sensitive tips of the fingers and toes from damage. Their appearance, texture and thickness may be significant in certain diseases.

Hair is present in nearly every part of the body except the palms of the hands and the soles of the feet. The hair grows out from a follicle in the dermis. It has a root and a shaft and varies in thickness.

Near the root of each hair is a small saccular gland. This is the *sebaceous gland* which produces an oily substance called *sebum*. Sebum is a lubricant for the hair and skin and makes the skin waterproof.

Sebum is also mildly antiseptic but it is greasy and there are millions of micro-organisms sticking to it. Because of this, some form of skin preparation must be performed before the skin is penetrated by a needle or scalpel, otherwise the organisms will enter the deeper structure and multiply. The skin preparation may consist of simply swabbing the skin with an antiseptic or shaving the hair and washing off the sebum with a detergent.

Attached to the hair follicles are small involuntary muscles called the *arrectores pilorum muscles*. When these muscles contract the hair will 'stand on end'. This happens in response to emotion, particularly fear, and also in cold conditions when the phenomenon is sometimes referred to as 'goose pimples'. The contraction of these muscles generates heat.

In the lower animals, the erection of the hair or feathers makes the animal look larger and fierce. A large amount of air is trapped in the fur, hair or feathers and this helps retain the body heat.

The skin questions

Diagrams—Questions 417–422

417–422. The skin

A. Epidermis		417
B. Dermis		418
C. Sebaceous gland		419
D. Sweat gland		420
E. Nerve endings		421
F. Blood vessels		422

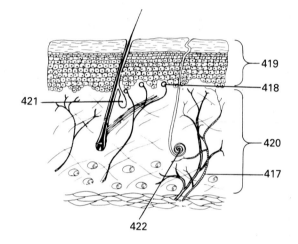

Questions 423–429 are of the multiple choice type.

423. **Which one of the following is not a function of the skin?**
    A. The excretion of waste
    B. The manufacture of vitamin A
    C. The regulation of body temperature
    D. It helps to maintain fluid balance.

    423

424. **The epidermis is composed of one of the following tissues. Which one?**
    A. Adipose tissue
    B. Elastic fibrous tissue
    C. Columnar epithelium
    D. Stratified squamous epithelium.

    424

425. **Which one of the following statements describes keratin? It is :**
    A. a type of protoplasm
    B. a horny substance
    C. the colouring matter in the skin
    D. the precursor of vitamin D.

    425

426. **The dermis is composed of one of the following tissues. Which one?**
    A. Adipose tissue
    B. Epithelial tissue
    C. White fibrous tissue
    D. Muscle tissue.

    426

427. **The epidermis contains one of the following :**
    A. ducts of glands
    B. blood vessels
    C. sebaceous glands
    D. sensory nerve endings.

    427

428. **Which one of the following substances is not present in sweat?**
    A. Calcium
    B. Potassium
    C. Sodium
    D. Water.

    428

429. **Which one of the following statements is true? A patient with pyrexia :**
    A. is in no danger if his temperature is below 40°C
    B. will sweat more as his temperature rises
    C. will sweat more as his temperature falls
    D. should be given extra blankets.

    429

Questions 430–465 are of the true/false type.

T | F

430–433. The dermis contains :
    430. ductless glands
    431. sebaceous glands
    432. lymphatic glands
    433. sweat glands.

434–437. Melanin :
    434. is present in the epidermis
    435. increases on exposure to the rays of the sun
    436. has a protective function
    437. makes the skin waterproof.

438–441. The arterioles in the skin :
    438. constrict in haemorrhage and shock
    439. constrict if the patient is afraid
    440. dilate in a cold bath
    441. dilate during exercise.

442–445. The sweat glands are :
    442. simple tubular glands
    443. coiled tubular glands
    444. saccular glands
    445. glands with ducts.

446–449. The excretion of sweat :
    446. is a continuous process
    447. helps to maintain electrolyte balance
    448. cools the body
    449. gets rid of the waste products of protein metabolism.

450–453. Body heat is gained by :
    450. shivering
    451. circulation of air at 30°C
    452. contraction of the arrectores pilorum muscles
    453. constriction of the arterioles.

454–457. Sebum :
    454. acts as a mild antiseptic
    455. is a waste product of metabolism
    456. is a trap for micro-organisms
    457. is secreted by the hair follicles.

458–461. **The arrectores pilorum muscles contract when the individual is :**   T | F

    458. exercising

    459. cold

    460. afraid

    461. in pain.

462–465. **A patient suffering from traumatic paraplegia :**

    462. feels pain over pressure points

    463. is liable to suffer occlusion of blood capillaries when pressure is unrelieved

    464. must be turned 2 hourly in order to protect the skin

    465. develops toughened skin over areas subjected to constant pressure.

8

The urinary system

The urinary system consists of the organs which regulate the amount of fluid in the body. In cold weather, less fluid is lost by sweating, so the urinary system produces more urine. In hot conditions, the amount of urine passed is reduced because more fluid is lost in sweat. If you drink a lot you pass more urine. All this is obvious, but the urinary system has a num-

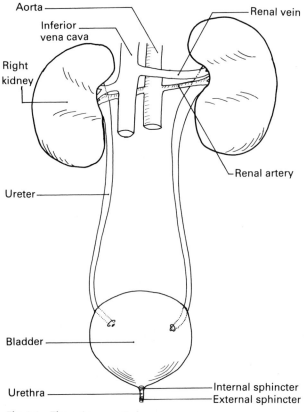

Fig. 8.1 The urinary system

ber of other functions. By regulating the volume of the body fluid it helps to maintain the blood pressure, the electrolyte content and the alkalinity of the blood. It is an excretory system and filters out urea and other waste substances.

Filtering the blood and the secretion of urine is the function of the *kidneys*. The *ureters, bladder* and *urethra* are concerned with the temporary storage and the discharge of the urine.

THE KIDNEYS

The kidneys are two bean-shaped organs which lie on the posterior abdominal wall behind the peritoneum on either side of the lumbar vertebrae. They are about 11 cm long and are embedded in a pad of fat which protects them and keeps them warm.

If a kidney is sliced longitudinally and examined, it will appear to have a solid portion and a hollow portion. The solid portion consists of thousands of minute tubules called *nephrons*. These nephrons are held together by connec-

tive tissue which contains blood and lymphatic vessels and nerves.

The hollow part of the kidney is the pelvis or upper expanded part of the ureter. This is where the urine collects before passing down into the bladder. It is shaped like a funnel and has several small funnel shaped structures called *calyces* round its upper edge.

The concave part of the kidney where the ureter leaves is called the *hilus*. This is where the renal artery enters and the renal vein and the lymphatic vessels leave. Covering the whole of the kidney is a loose bag of elastic fibrous tissue called the renal *capsule*. Attached to the upper pole of each kidney are the *adrenal glands* (see p. 171).

THE MICROSCOPIC STRUCTURE OF THE KIDNEY

The solid part of the kidney consists of two parts. The outer part is called the *cortex* and is brownish-red in colour. The middle part, or *medulla*, is paler and consists of pyramid-shaped structures. The apices of the pyramids enter the calyces (see Fig. 8.2).

The nephrons

The nephrons are twisted tubules made of very specialised epithelial cells, and it is here that the urine is manufactured. Each nephron starts as a little cup-shaped filter called the *glomerular capsule*. The second part of the nephron is a *convoluted tubule* which, with the glomerular capsule, lies in the cortex. From this first convoluting tubule a straight tube passes down into the medulla. This is the *loop of Henle*. It makes a 'U' turn and loops back into the cortex where the *second convoluted tubule* lies. This tubule ends in a straight *collecting tubule* which passes through the medulla to open into the calyces (Fig. 8.3). Entering each glomerular capsule is a branch of the renal artery. This vessel forms loops of capillaries called the glomerulus. The pressure of the blood in these capillaries pushes water and other substances through the glomerular capsule into the first convoluted tubule. The cap-

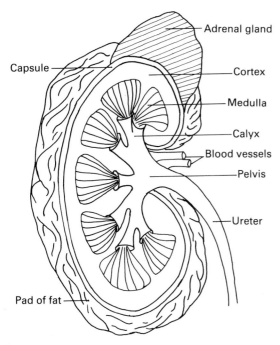

Fig. 8.2 A section through a kidney

Adrenal gland

Capsule

Cortex

Medulla

Calyx

Blood vessels

Pelvis

Ureter

Pad of fat

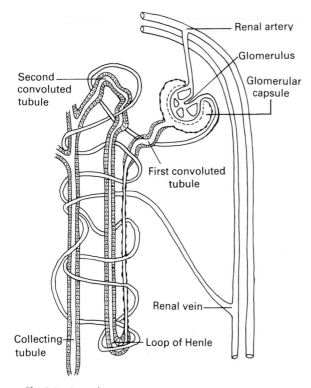

Second convoluted tubule

Renal artery

Glomerulus

Glomerular capsule

First convoluted tubule

Renal vein

Collecting tubule

Loop of Henle

Fig. 8.3 A nephron

sule acts as a filter and holds back albumen and blood cells. These substances continue on through the capillary network which leaves the glomerulus and winds round the convoluting tubules. The capillaries become the venules which join up to form the renal vein.

THE FORMATION OF URINE

The fluid which passes through the glomerular filter is called the filtrate as it is not yet urine. It contains glucose and amino acids as well as mineral salts and urea. Nutrients do not normally appear in urine. They are reabsorbed into the capillaries with water from the convoluted tubules. The cells of the convoluted tubules secrete toxins, drugs and other foreign substances into the filtrate. Most drugs given to patients are excreted in the urine. That is why they must be given regularly, as prescribed, if the correct level in the blood is to be maintained. A missed dose of medicine means a period of time without treatment.

The fluid which flows from the collecting tubules is now urine. Urine consists of 96% water, 2% urea and 2% mineral salts—mainly sodium chloride. It contains the things the body does not want. These include urea, the waste product of protein metabolism, the amount of which depends on the individual's diet. Excess sodium chloride is also excreted to balance the salt taken in food over and above that required to maintain the correct osmotic pressure of the body fluids. In addition, small quantities of other minerals and substances derived from protein, such as uric acid, are present.

Urine is a pale amber coloured fluid with a specific gravity of between 1015 and 1025. It is normally an acid fluid. The excretion of acid salts maintains the alkalinity of the blood.

The secretion of urine by the kidneys is controlled by the *antidiuretic hormone* from the *pituitary gland*. (see p. 169). The pituitary gland is influenced by the osmotic pressure of the blood. The amount of urine passed by a healthy individual in one day is between 1000 and 1500 ml.

Examination of the urine is an important aid to diagnosis. Glucose is present if the blood sugar level is too high, as in diabetes mellitus. Too much sugar in the blood is called hyperglycaemia. Acetone may also be present in the urine of a diabetic patient. In nephritis, which is inflammation of the kidneys, the damaged nephrons allow albumen and blood through the glomerular capsule into the urine. Bile is present if the patient is jaundiced and bile is circulating in the blood stream, instead of being excreted in the faeces. There are, of course, other abnormal substances found in the urine, but many of these can only be discovered on microscopic examination.

THE URETERS

The ureters are continuous with the kidney pelvis. They leave the kidneys along with the renal veins at the hilus. The ureters carry the urine down to the bladder for storage and the renal veins carry the filtered blood into the vena cava.

The ureters are muscular tubes about 30 cm in length. They are lined with mucous membrane and are covered with fibrous tissue. They pass down through the abdomen into the pelvis where they enter the bladder. The muscular contractions of the ureter propels the urine down into the bladder by persitalsis. This is the reason why a patient nursed flat on his back can still pass urine, although the kidneys lie at a lower level then the bladder. This type of immobilisation is one of the causes of *renal calculi*. These are stones which may be formed from crystals of calcium salts in a sluggish urinary system. Renal *colic* is the agonising pain which results from spasms of the ureters as the stone is passed along. These patients should be given copious fluids to drink and their position should be changed as often as possible to prevent the formation of calculi.

THE BLADDER

When the bladder is empty it is a pelvic organ, but as it fills up with urine it stretches and can be palpated in the abdomen above the symphysis pubis. In the female it lies in front of the uterus which it helps to support.

The bladder is made of involuntary muscle tissue. It is lined with transitional epithelium which is smooth when the bladder is full and in folds when the bladder is empty. It is covered on its upper surface by the peritoneum.

The ureters enter the bladder at the back the urethra leaves below at the neck of the bladder.

The bladder acts as a reservoir for urine and will hold up to 200 to 300 ml quite comfortably.

THE URETHRA

At the neck of the bladder where the urethra leaves, is a sphincter muscle. This is the internal sphincter which, like the rest of the bladder, is controlled by the autonomic nervous system. The female urethra is a short tube about 4 cm long. Its structure is similar to the

bladder. The opening to the outside is guarded by the external sphincter muscle which is under the control of the will. The male urethra is much longer and is described as part of the male reproductive system (see p. 181).

MICTURITION

Micturition is the act of passing urine. When about 300 ml of urine have collected in the bladder the pressure will stimulate the sensory nerves in the bladder wall. The individual becomes aware of the need to empty the bladder but can control this desire for a limited period of time until it is convenient. In infancy, micturition is a reflex action and there is no control from the brain.

The night nurse in a geriatric ward should always offer a bed pan if a patient is restless and not sleeping. The cause is often a desire to micturate.

When micturition occurs, the bladder wall contracts. The anterior abdominal wall also contracts and puts pressure on the bladder. The internal sphincter slowly opens, the external sphincter relaxes and the bladder is emptied.

Retention of urine in the bladder occurs when there is a brain or spinal cord lesion, some form of obstruction in the urethra, or after an operation. Post-operative retention occurs most frequently after pelvic operations when the bladder has been handled. The bladder will stretch until it holds as much as 1 to 1½ litres of urine. The patient cannot pass urine; he becomes very distressed and suffers severe pain. This is usually a nursing problem. Help can be given by getting the patient out of bed into a more natural position for micturition if this is possible. Privacy, sympathy and understanding are often all that is necessary. Sometimes the bladder must be catheterised. As the bladder is a sterile organ, this must be a sterile procedure. The introduction of microorganisms into the bladder causes *cystitis* which is a painful and distressing condition.

Retention with *overflow* occurs in unconscious patients. The bladder is full, the external sphincter relaxes and allows a little urine to escape. The patient is continually wet and great care must be taken to protect the skin as it will break down if allowed to remain in contact with wet sheets.

Incontinence is the involuntary passing of urine, and may be the result of weakness of the sphincter. There are many causes of incontinence. Elderly women often suffer from stress incontinence when urine is voided following coughing, sneezing or laughing. This can be very embarrasing.

Oedema is a sign of kidney disease. The amount of fluid in the tissues is increased as the diseased kidneys cannot secrete enough to maintain the fluid balance. The oedema appears as a puffy swelling of the face and ankles. *Diuretics* are drugs used to increase the amount of urine formed by the kidneys.

Anuria means that the secretion of urine by the kidneys is suppressed. No urine is passed, the amount of urea in the blood increases and the patient suffers from *uraemia* which will be fatal if not treated. In renal failure, the blood must be filtered mechanically by using a kidney machine. This is called dialysis and may be followed by a kidney transplantation.

Urinary system questions

Diagrams—Questions 466–483

466–471. The urinary system

A. Inferior vena cava
B. Aorta
C. Renal arteries
D. Renal veins
E. Ureter
F. Urethra.

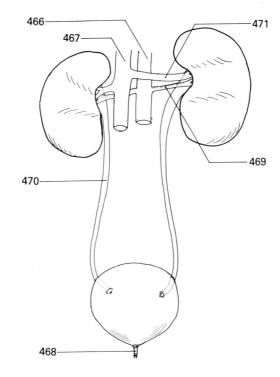

466
467
468
469
470
471

472–477. A section through the kidney

A. Cortex
B. Medulla
C. Capsule
D. Pelvis
E. Calyx
F. Ureter

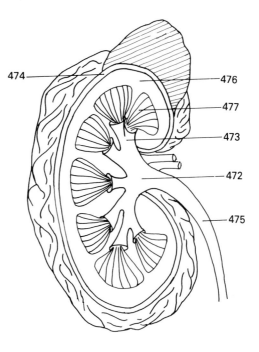

472
473
474
475
476
477

478–483. A nephron

- A. Glomerular capsule
- B. Glomerulus
- C. Second convoluting tubule
- D. Loop of Henle
- E. Collecting tubule
- F. Renal artery

478
479
480
481
482
483

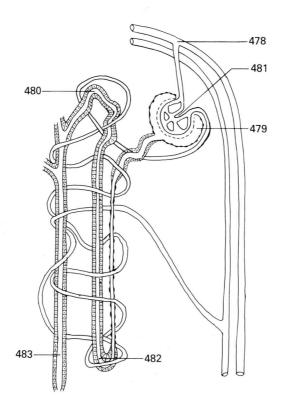

Questions 484–491 are of the multiple choice type.

484. Which one of the following enters the kidney at the hilus?
    A. Ureter
    B. Renal vein
    C. Renal artery
    D. Lymphatic vessel.

484

485. Which one of the following is the part of the kidney which acts as a filter?
    A. Loop of Henle
    B. Glomerular capsule
    C. The collecting tubule
    D. The pelvis.

485

486. Which one of the following is not part of a nephron?
    A. The calyx
    B. The convoluted tubule
    C. The loop of Henle
    D. The collecting tubule.

486

487. Which one of the following substances does not pass through the glomerular capsule?
    A. Mineral salts
    B. Glucose
    C. Protein
    D. Urea.

487

488. A healthy individual will pass approximately one of the following amounts of urine per day. Which one?
    A. 500 millilitres
    B. 1250 millilitres
    C. 2000 millilitres
    D. 2500 millilitres.

488

489. Which one of the following is correct? Normal urine :
    A. is alkaline
    B. has a specific gravity of 1050
    C. contains 75% water
    D. contains 2% sodium chloride.

489

490. The urinary bladder :
    A. concentrates urine
    B. stores urine
    C. manufactures urine
    D. secretes urine.

490

491. **In nephritis the urine contains :**   491
   A. albumen
   B. bile
   C. acetone
   D. glucose.

Questions 492–507 are of the true/false type.

492–495. The kidney :

    492. is approximately 11
         centimetres long
    493. lies behind the peritoneum
    494. lies in the iliac regions of the
         abdomen
    495. contains no lymphatic vessels.

496–499. The glomerulus :

    496. is cup-shaped
    497. is a collection of capillaries
    498. is a lymphatic node
    499. is part of the renal circulation.

500–503. The ureters :

    500. are continuations of the nephrons
    501. are made of voluntary muscle tissue
    502. move the urine along by peristalsis
    503. commence at the kidney pelvis.

504–507. During micturition :

    504. the abdominal wall contracts
    505. the bladder wall relaxes
    506. the internal sphincter opens
    507. the external sphincter opens by reflex action.

Questions 508–510 are of the matching items type.

508–510. From the list on the left select the statement which defines the conditions on the right.

A. The kidney is not producing urine   508. Retention | 508

B. The bladder empties involuntarily   509. Renal colic | 509

C. The sphincter muscle may be in spasm   510. Anuria. | 510

D. Infection has entered the bladder

E. The ureter is in spasm causing pain

9

The nervous system

The nervous system is the most complex system in the body. Without a nerve supply, the organs of the body cannot work. Life without a brain is impossible.

One of the first lessons a nurse must learn is to be observant and to use her brain. Being observant does not mean simply keeping her eyes open. The night nurse writing her report about a very ill patient does not describe only what she sees but what she has heard, felt and smelled. She uses all her sense organs with the possible exception of taste. The eyes, the ears, the nose and the skin must all play a part in observation. The report will describe that she saw the patient sleeping but she also heard his hacking cough, felt his hot dry skin and smelled his bad breath. All these facts are fed into the sister's brain. Because of her experience sister can immediately sum up the patient's condition.

Life is one big collection of experiences. We are aware of sights, sounds, tastes, smells and pain. We can also feel things, their texture, shape and temperature. The brain receives these sensations and stores the information as memory. As the individual is exposed to new experiences, he stores the new knowledge and adjusts his memory. He learns facts and what to do with these facts. He thinks and reasons and so develops an intellect.

The young infant has no reasoning ability. All his actions are reflex actions. He is guided by his instincts. He yells when he is hungry, cries when he is hurt and empties his bladder and bowel when they are full. Gradually his

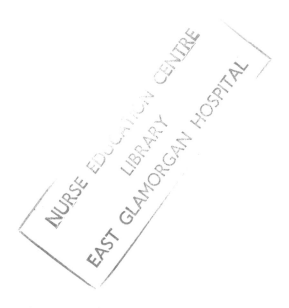

nervous system develops and, with his mother's guidance, he learns some control. He also learns about his surroundings. He sees an orange; he is allowed to feel it; he learns that when the peel comes off it has a special smell. He is given a piece to taste and so eventually the whole picture of an orange is stored in his brain. This process of learning and of memory modification continues throughout life.

Because of his experiences the child begins to get curious. If this curiosity is to be satisfied he must learn to control his limbs; to sit up; reach out and eventually walk. The coordination of muscles, which is part of the controlling function of the brain, is of vital importance to his development.

The structure and function of the nervous system is very complicated and not completely understood. It can be divided into three parts:
  the central nervous system
  the peripheral nervous system
  the autonomic nervous system.

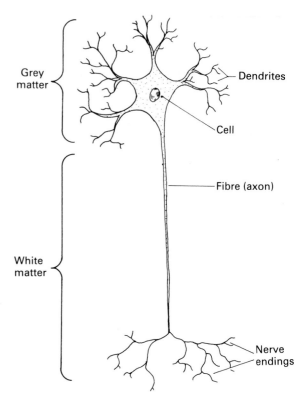

Fig. 9.1 A neuron

THE CENTRAL NERVOUS SYSTEM

The central nervous system consists of the brain and spinal cord. These are made of nervous tissue which is sometimes described as *grey* and *white matter*. If you look at a section of the brain you will see that it is grey on the outside and white on the inside. A microscopic examination will show that the grey matter consists of cells and the white matter is made up of fibres.

A cell and its fibres is called a *neuron*. There are billions of neurons making up the nervous system.

Neurons

Each neuron is a nerve cell with projections of its protoplasm forming *dendrites* and one long *axon*. The dendrites are short, branched fibres and each cell has several dendrites. Axons leave the grey matter and become the fibres of the white matter. All axons have a covering called a *neurilemma* and most have a fatty

sheath which acts as an insulating material. This is called the *myelin sheath*.

There are two types of neuron—*sensory* and *motor*. Nerve impulses which resemble little electric currents pass along the axon. In a sensory neuron the impulse passes towards the cell, and in a motor neuron it passes away from the cell.

Sensory neurons start as nerve endings situated in the sensory organs. Impulses recording sensations are carried from these organs into the cell and eventually to the brain.

Motor neurons end in muscles. Impulses pass from the cell in the brain out to the muscles to initiate movement.

The brain

The brain consists of three parts:
  the cerebrum
  the brain stem
  the cerebellum.

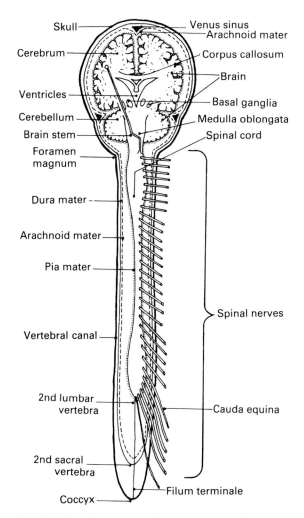

Skull

Cerebrum

Ventricles

Cerebellum

Brain stem

Foramen magnum

Dura mater

Arachnoid mater

Pia mater

Vertebral canal

2nd lumbar vertebra

2nd sacral vertebra

Coccyx

Venus sinus

Arachnoid mater

Corpus callosum

Brain

Basal ganglia

Medulla oblongata

Spinal cord

Spinal nerves

Cauda equina

Filum terminale

Fig. 9.2 Central nervous system

The cerebrum

The cerebrum is the largest part of the brain. It occupies most of the skull. It consists of two hemispheres which are joined by a bridge of white matter called the *corpus callosum*. Under the corpus callosum are the lateral *ventricles*. These are cavities in the brain which contain *cerebrospinal fluid*. The cerebrospinal fluid comes from a collection of blood capillaries in the roofs of the ventricles. This fluid circulates round the brain and spinal cord protecting and nourishing them.

The surface of the cerebrum is called the *cerebral cortex*. It consists of billions of packed nerve cells, each with its own axon. These axons pass downwards through the lower parts of the brain into the brain stem and some continue down into the spinal cord. In the brain stem the axons cross each other so that those from the left hemisphere cross to the right side of the cord and vice versa.

The cerebral cortex has a wrinkled appearance like a walnut. The folds increase the surface area of the grey matter. It is divided into lobes by fissures. The lobes take their names from the bones beneath which they lie. Therfore each hemisphere has a frontal, parietal, temporal and occipital lobe.

The functions of the cerebrum are to initiate and control the movements of the skeletal muscles and to receive impulses from the sensory organs. There are groups of cells which are the emotional, thinking, reasoning and re-

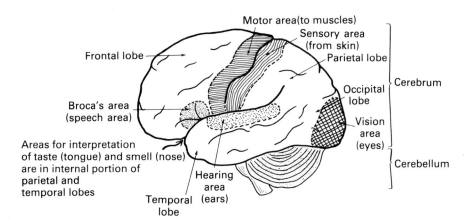

Motor area(to muscles)

Sensory area (from skin)

Parietal lobe

Frontal lobe

Occipital lobe

Cerebrum

Broca's area (speech area)

Vision area (eyes)

Cerebellum

Areas for interpretation of taste (tongue) and smell (nose) are in internal portion of parietal and temporal lobes

Hearing area (ears)

Temporal lobe

Fig. 9.3 The cerebral cortex

membering centres. The grey matter of the cortex has been mapped out and certain functions attributed to the different lobes.

The areas concerned with movement are in the frontal lobes. They are called the motor areas. The areas concerned with the skin sensation are in the parietal lobes, lying alongside the motor areas but separated from them by deep fissures. The areas responsible for sight are in the occipital lobes and the hearing and smell areas are in the temporal lobes. The area for taste is thought to be in the sensory area in the parietal lobes. In the frontal lobes there are so-called silent areas which are thought to be concerned with thought, emotion, behaviour and intelligence.

The speech area is called Broca's area and is in the frontal lobe. It is the centre concerned with the movements required for speech. The speech centre is active in the dominant hemisphere which is the left one in a right-handed person. If a patient who has had a stroke is paralysed down the right side his speech is most likely to be affected because his cerebro-vascular accident will have been in the left hemisphere. These patients know what they want to say but cannot say it. They require a great deal of support and understanding. The relatives as well as the nurse must learn to have patience, to anticipate the patient's needs and to teach him new ways to communicate.

The deep layers of the cerebral cortex consist of white matter with the exception of some groups of cells or ganglia near the base of the cerebrum. These are the *basal ganglia*, the *thalamus* and the *hypothalamus*. The basal ganglia is concerned with the co-ordination of muscle action. The thalamus relays sensory impulses to the brain for interpretation. The hypothalamus is associated with the pituitary gland and its hormones.

The brain stem

The brain stem connects the cerebrum to the spinal cord. It consists of three parts: the midbrain, the pons varolii and the medulla oblongata.

The *midbrain* is where the fibres from the two hemispheres come together. They lie in two bundles and pass under the *pons varolii* which is a bridge of fibres connecting the two hemispheres of the cerebellum.

The *medulla oblongata* is continuous with the spinal cord and consists of white matter on the outside and grey matter on the inside. This is where the fibres cross over to the opposite side. The grey matter controls the heart, the blood vessels and respiration. The *cardiac centre* controls the rate and force of the heart. The *respiratory centre* controls the rate and depth of respiration. The *vaso-motor* centre controls the muscular walls of the small blood vessels, causing vasoconstriction or vasodilation to occur.

There are also *reflex centres* in the medulla oblongata. These initiate coughing, sneezing and vomiting when something is irritating the respiratory tract or the stomach.

The cerebellum

The cerebellum is the hindbrain. It is situated at the back, beneath the occipital lobe of the cerebrum. Like the cerebrum it has grey matter on the outside and white matter inside. It consists of two hemispheres joined by a bridge of fibres called the *vermis*.

The cerebellum is connected to the cerebrum, the brain stem and the spinal cord. Its functions are co-ordination of muscle movement, balance and maintaining the tone of the muscles so that they are ready for immediate action. Watch a child learning to ride a bicycle and think of the functions of the cerebellum.

The blood supply to the brain

The carotid arteries and the vertebral arteries supply blood to the brain. These arteries branch and join up again, forming a circle of arteries at the base of the brain called the *Circle of Willis*. From here smaller *cerebral* arteries branch off to supply each region of the brain.

Blood returns from the brain to the superior

vena cava by the *jugular veins*. The venous blood collects in channels called the *venous sinuses* which lie between the layers of the dura mater (see p. 145). From these venous sinuses the blood drains into the jugular veins.

The spinal cord

The spinal cord is a continuation of the brain stem. It lies in the vertebral canal extending from the foremen magnum to between the first and second lumbar vertebrae. It is cylindrical, approximately 45 cm long and about the same thickness as the little finger.

The spinal cord consists of grey matter on the inside and white matter on the outside. The grey matter continues through the whole length of the spinal cord rather like the lettering in a stick of rock. In section it is roughly the shape of the letter 'H'. There is a tiny central canal which is continuous with the ventricles of the brain and contains cerebrospinal fluid.

From the cells in the grey matter come the fibres which form the spinal or peripheral nerves. The anterior horns of the grey matter (see Fig. 9.4) contain the cells of the motor neurons which supply the muscles. The posterior horns contain the cells of the sensory neurons which supply the skin. The beginnings of the axons from these cells are called the motor and sensory roots. They form the roots of the spinal nerves. The roots come together just as they leave the vertebral canal, where they are bound in a common sheath to form a nerve. Injury to a nerve will, therefore, cause loss of sensation as well as of movement.

The white matter of the spinal cord consists of nerve fibres or axons lying in anterior, posterior and lateral columns. These are the fibres which form the sensory and motor pathways to and from the brain.

The sensory and motor pathways

Consider what happens when you touch something unpleasant and decide to withdraw your hand. The sensory nerve endings in the skin are stimulated by the object. An impluse

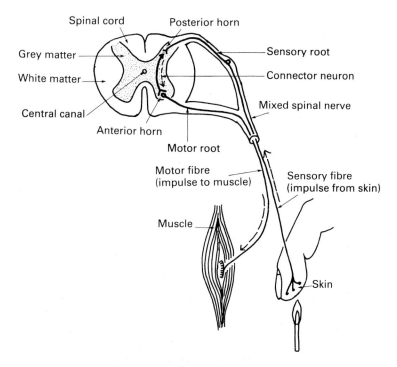

Fig. 9.4 Diagrammatic section of spinal cord to show reflex action

passes up the peripheral nerve into the posterior horns of the spinal cord. From here the impulse is transmitted to the white matter where it travels up another sensory neuron to the thalamus where the sensation is felt but only crudely. From the thalamus, the sensation is relayed by another neuron to the sensory area of the cortex of the brain where the fine sensation is interpreted. There are, therefore, three different lots of sensory neurons involved before you can feel the exact temperature, shape and texture of an object.

To withdraw the hand, impulses pass down from the brain through two groups of motor neurons. The *upper motor neurons* have their cells in the cerebral cortex and their axons in the brain, brain stem and spinal cord. The impulses pass from the brain down the cord to the level at which the spinal nerve leaves. If the nerve is supplying muscle of the lower limbs the axon will continue to the end of the cord. When it is the upper limb you wish to move, the axons will stop in the neck. The impulses will then be transmitted to the cells in the anterior horn of the grey matter and a second or *lower motor neuron* will convey the impulse to the muscles by the peripheral nerves. The muscles will contract and produce the required movement.

Reflex action

There are occasions when the movements of voluntary muscles are not controlled by the brain. In the grey matter of the spinal cord, between the cells of the anterior and posterior horns, are small connector neurons which will transmit an impulse straight from the skin to muscles (see Fig. 9.4). This is called reflex action and it occurs if you touch something which is dangerous. You will have withdrawn your hand before you are aware of unacceptable heat or pain.

When the doctor is examining a patient he may want to test his reflexes. Fortunately, this can be done without causing pain. A tendon hammer is used to tap the patellar tendon when the knee is flexed and relaxed. The result is an uncontrolled contraction of the quadriceps muscle and the knee jerks into extension.

Although reflex action is mainly protective in function, you can if you exert a great deal of willpower control the action. Consider your reaction if you are having a meal on your own and you put a spoonfull of boiling soup into your mouth. You will spit it out just as a baby will do if it is fed pudding which is too hot. Think of the same circumstance in a crowded restaurant. Having been taught that it is rude to spit out your food in front of other people you control this reflex action. You will swallow the soup and burn your tongue whilst doing so!

The meninges

The meninges are protective coverings for the brain and the spinal cord. There are three membranes. The outer one lines the skull and vertebral canal as far as the second sacral vertebra and is called the *dura mater*. The other two lie between the dura mater and the brain and spinal cord. They are the *arachnoid mater* and the *pia mater*.

The dura mater

The dura mater consists of two layers of tough fibrous tissue. The two layers are close together except where the inner layer dips down between the hemispheres of the cerebrum and between the cerebellum and the cerebrum (see Fig. 9.2). At these points the dura mater forms the venous sinuses, the channels into which the venous blood drains (see p. 142).

The arachnoid mater

The arachnoid mater, so called because it resembles a spider's web, is a fine covering of serous membrane which lies under the dura mater. It is separated from the dura mater by a potential space called the subdural space. It covers the brain and spinal cord and extends down to the second sacral vertebra.

The pia mater

The pia mater is a fine membrane consisting of minute blood vessels held together by areolar tissue. The pia mater covers the brain and dips down between the convolutions and fissures on the brain surface. It covers the spinal cord and continues down as a thread-like structure from the end of the cord to fuse with the sacrum. This thread is called the *filum terminale*, and it helps to anchor the cord preventing unnecessary movement.

Between the arachnoid mater and the pia mater is a space called the *subarachnoid space*. This space contains *cerebrospinal fluid*, a clear watery fluid containing mineral salts and traces of protein and glucose. The fluid is secreted into the *ventricles* of the brain from capillaries in the roof of each ventricle. There are four ventricles. The two lateral ventricles have already been discussed. The third ventricle lies below them and the fourth lies between the cerebellum and the pons varolii.

Cerebrospinal fluid circulates from the ventricles round the brain and spinal cord, acting as a water cushion or shock absorber. It protects these delicate structures from contact injury with the hard skull and the walls of the vertebral canal.

The subarachnoid space below the end of the cord contains cerebrospinal fluid and the roots of the nerves which supply the lower limbs. This collection of roots resembles the coarse hair of a horse's tail, which is why it is called the *cauda equina*.

A *lumbar puncture* is the introduction of a needle into the subarachnoid space in order to draw off some of the cerebrospinal fluid. This procedure is performed for diagnostic reasons, to introduce drugs and occasionally to relieve irritation. A patient being prepared for lumbar puncture must be placed in such a position that the spine is in complete flexion. This opens up the space between the vertebrae to allow the needle to penetrate the meninges. The needle is introduced below the level of the third lumbar vertebra to prevent injury to the spinal cord itself.

THE PERIPHERAL NERVOUS SYSTEM

The peripheral nervous system consists of the nerves which leave the brain stem and spinal cord. There are twelve pairs of *cranial nerves* supplying the structures above the neck. The trunk and limbs are supplied by 31 pairs of *spinal nerves*.

The cranial nerves

There are twelve pairs of cranial nerves leaving the brain stem. Four pairs of these nerves supply the sensory organs in the skull.

The *olfactory* nerve is the nerve of smell.

The *glossopharangeal* nerve is the nerve of taste.

The *auditory* nerve is the nerve of hearing.

The *optic* nerve is the nerve of sight.

Three pairs of cranial nerves supply the muscles which move the eyeballs, an important part of facial expression. Facial expression also includes movement of the facial muscles which are supplied by the facial nerve. The trigeminal nerve supplies the skin of the face and the muscles of mastication. Other cranial nerves supply the muscles which move the head and the tongue.

The *vagus* nerve is the only cranial nerve which passes into the trunk. This is a sensory and motor nerve which supplies the organs of the thorax and abdomen. It is part of the autonomic nervous system.

The spinal nerves

The spinal nerves pass out of the vertebral canal, one pair emerging below each vertebra and one pair emerging between the cranium and the first cervical vertebra.
This gives:

eight pairs of cervical nerves
twelve pairs of thoracic nerves
five pairs of lumbar nerves
five pairs of sacral nerves
one pair of coccygeal nerves.

The lumbar, sacral and coccygeal nerves pass straight down from the end of the spinal cord to reach their respective exit foramina.

The roots of these nerves form the cauda equina (see Fig. 9.2).

Each nerve contains motor and sensory fibres. They come from the cells in the anterior and posterior horns of the grey matter of the spinal cord. As these fibres leave the cord they form the motor and sensory roots. The roots come together as they leave the vertebral canal to form the spinal nerves. A spinal nerve consists of bundles of nerve fibres wrapped up in connective tissue for protection. Before the nerves reach the limbs they form networks rather like railway junctions. Each of these networks is called a *plexus*.

The nerves from the *cervical plexus* supply the skin and the muscles of the neck.

The nerves from the *brachial plexus* supply the upper limbs. The brachial plexus lies in the axilla and has five branches. The *radial* nerve which supplies the extensor muscles of the wrist and fingers has already been mentioned because it can be damaged so easily by careless handling of an unconscious patient (see p. 29). The *median* nerve supplies the flexor muscles of the wrist and fingers and thumb.

The *ulnar* nerve supplies the muscles of the hand and the *axillary* nerve supplies the muscles which move the shoulders. The *musculocutaneous* nerve supplies the biceps muscle which flexes the elbow. These nerves also supply some part of the skin of the upper limbs.

The thoracic nerves do not form a plexus but pass round the chest wall protected by the ribs. They supply the muscles and skin of the thorax and abdomen.

The *lumbar plexus* has two main branches. The *femoral* nerve supplies the quadriceps muscle which extends the knee, and the *obturator* nerve supplies the adductor muscles of the hip.

The *sacral plexus* has one large branch, the *sciatic* nerve, and some smaller branches, the *gluteal* nerves. The gluteal nerves supply the muscles of the hip. The sciatic nerve is the nerve which can be damaged by an incorrectly given intramuscular injection into the buttock. This nerve supplies the hamstring muscles which flex the knee and all the muscles below the knee which act on the ankle joint and toes. The *common peroneal nerve*, a branch of the

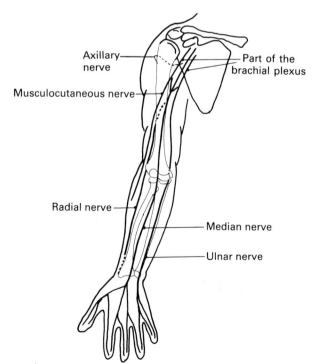

Fig. 9.5 The peripheral nerves of the upper limb

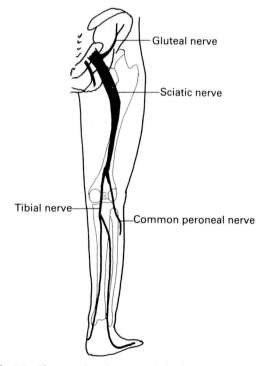

Fig. 9.6 The peripheral nerves of the lower limb

sciatic nerve, has already been referred to (p. 54). Injury to this nerve at the point where it winds round the lateral aspect of the knee may be the cause of dropped foot. It is pressure on this nerve which gives you 'pins and needles' if you sit too long with your knees crossed. The skin of the lower limbs and pelvis is supplied by nerves from the lumbar and sacral plexuses.

THE AUTONOMIC NERVOUS SYSTEM

The autonomic nervous system is the part of the nervous system which supplies the involuntary muscle tissue of the body. It controls the movements of the internal organs and the secretions of the glands.

There are two parts to the autonomic nervous system. The *sympathetic nervous system* and the *parasympathetic nervous system*. The autonomic nerve cells are situated in the brain stem and spinal cord. The axons leave the spinal cord and brain stem with the peripheral nerves.

Before being distributed to the various organs, the fibres of the *sympathetic* nervous system enter a chain of *ganglia* which lie on either side of the vertebral column.

The *parasympathetic* nervous system consists of the *vagus* nerve and autonomic fibres which accompany the sacral nerves.

The parts of the autonomic nervous system have opposing effects on the body. They both send out weak impulses to the organs and glands maintaining normal activity. However, in stressful situations the sympathetic impulses become stronger and the organs and glands react to the situation. The parasympathetic nerves will take over when the stressful situation has passed and the functions of the organs return to normal.

If you are very apprehensive, terrified or making a really great effort, your heart will beat faster. The blood vessels to the coronary and skeletal muscles and to the bronchioles will dilate. The liver will produce more glucose from glycogen. The small arterioles in the skin will constrict and your blood pressure will rise. You will go white but your muscles and your brain will be getting more oxygen and glucose and you will be prepared for both physical and mental action. At the same time, the pupils of your eyes will dilate, your hair will stand on end and the sweat glands will produce more sweat. Meanwhile the secretion of the digestive juices and the movements of the stomach and bowel are inhibited, your mouth becomes dry and you feel sick. This is the effect of the sympathetic nervous system preparing you for whatever action is desirable. Will you stay and fight or will you turn and run?

After the stressful situation is over, the parasympathetic nervous system returns things to normal. The digestive organs receive more blood, the glands increase their secretions and the excretory organs begin to function again. The heart beat is decreased, the blood pressure falls and peace is restored.

A worried and upset patient will not be physiologically ready to digest his food. The nurse must try to relieve him of his anxieties before presenting him with his meal.

Nervous system questions

Diagrams—Questions 511–550

511–514. A neuron
    A. Dendrite
    B. Axon
    C. Nucleus
    D. Cell

511
512
513
514

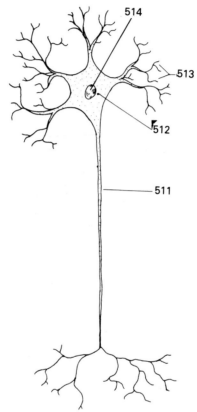

515–526. Central nervous system

A.	Cerebrum	515
B.	Cerebellum	516
C.	Ventricles	517
D.	Medulla oblongata	518
E.	Spinal cord	519
F.	Cauda equina	520
G.	Filum terminale	521
H.	Pia mater	522
I.	Dura mater	523
J.	Foramen magnum	524
K.	A thoracic nerve	525
L.	A lumbar nerve	526

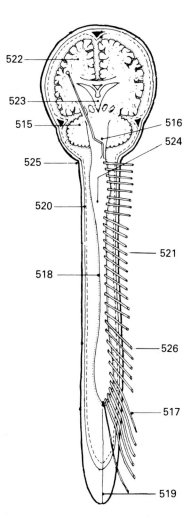

527–535. The cerebral cortex

A. Frontal lobe	527
B. Parietal lobe	528
C. Temporal lobe	529
D. Occipital lobe	530
E. Motor area	531
F. Sensory area	532
G. Vision area	533
H. Hearing area	534
I. Speech area	535

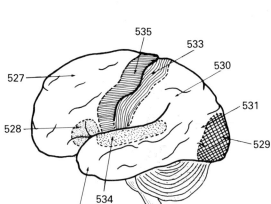

536–542. Section through spinal cord

A. Posterior root	536
B. Anterior root	537
C. Posterior horn	538
D. Connector neuron	539
E. Spinal nerve	540
F. Motor nerve ending	541
G. Central canal	542

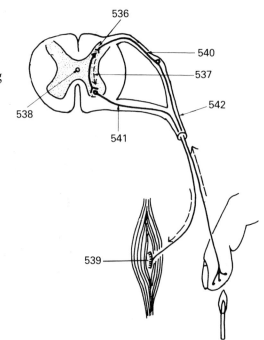

543–546. Peripheral nerves
   A. Brachial plexus
   B. Radial nerve
   C. Median nerve
   D. Ulnar nerve

543
544
545
546

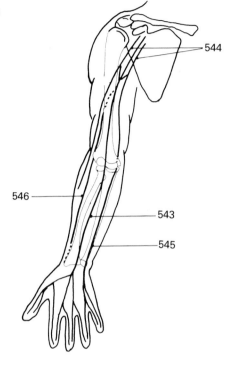

547–550. A. Sciatic nerve
   B. Common peroneal nerve
   C. Gluteal nerve
   D. Tibial nerve

547
548
549
550

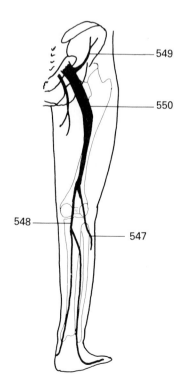

Questions 551–555 are of the multiple choice type.

551. The unit of the nervous system is a :

A. nephron
B. neutron
C. neuron
D. nerve.

552. Which one of the following is the fatty covering of an axon?

A. Neuroglia
B. Neurilemma
C. Myelin sheath
D. Adipose tissue.

553. The venous sinuses of the brain lie between the :

A. dura mater and the skull
B. inner and outer layers of the dura mater
C. arachnoid mater and the pia mater
D. dura mater and the arachnoid mater.

554. Which one of the following is a function of the sympathetic nervous system? Constriction of the :

A. bronchioles
B. coronary artery
C. skin arterioles
D. pupils.

555. Which one of the following is a function of the parasympathetic nervous system?

A. The heart beat is increased
B. The blood pressure rises
C. There is an increase in the flow of saliva
D. The secretion of gastric juice decreases.

Questions 556–587 are of the true/false type.

T | F

556–559. The central nervous system controls :
  556. growth
  557. the movement of the skeleton
  558. the flow of gastric juice
  559. peristalsis.

560–563. From which of the following arteries does the brain receive its blood supply?
  560. Carotid
  561. Facial
  562. Subclavian
  563. Vertebral.

564–567. The cerebrum :
  564. has two hemispheres
  565. is composed entirely of grey matter
  566. is divided into six lobes
  567. is protected by cerebrospinal fluid.

568–571. The spinal cord :
  568. is about 45 cm long
  569. extends to the end of the vertebral canal
  570. contains a central canal
  571. has grey matter on the outside.

572–575. The cranial nerves :
  572. lie entirely within the skull
  573. number 12 pairs
  574. have their roots in the spinal cord
  575. are all motor nerves.

576–579. The spinal nerves :
  576. number 32 pairs
  577. are all mixed nerves
  578. form plexuses
  579. supply the internal organs.

580–583. The brachial plexus :   T   F

     580. lies in the axilla
     581. has two branches
     582. supplies the chest wall
     583. supplies the upper limb.

584–587. The branches of the sacral plexus form the :

     584. femoral nerve
     585. gluteal nerve
     586. obturator nerve
     587. sciatic nerve.

Questions 588–605 are of the matching items type.

588–590. From the list on the left select the function associated with each lobe of the cerebrum listed on the right.

A. Hearing
B. Sight
C. Movement
D. Touch
E. Smell

588. Frontal
589. Parietal
590. Occipital.

588
589
590

591–593. From the list on the left select the statement which relates to each part of the brain stem listed on the right.

A. Connects the cerebellar hemispheres
B. Contains the hypothalamus
C. Is where the fibres cross
D. Contains Broca's area
E. Is the uppermost part of the brain stem

591. Midbrain
592. Pons varolii
593. Medulla oblongata.

591
592
593

594–596. From the list on the left select the statement which describes each of the structures listed on the right.

A. Lines the skull and vertebral canal
B. Consists of serous membrane
C. Secretes cerebrospinal fluid
D. Forms the filum terminale
E. Forms the cauda equina

594. Arachnoid mater
595. Pia mater
596. Dura mater.

594
595
596

597–599. From the list on the left select the contents of the parts of the spinal cord listed on the right.

A. Motor fibres only
B. Motor cells
C. Sensory and motor fibres
D. Sensory cells
E. Sympathetic nerves

597. Anterior horns
598. Posterior horns
599. Columns of white matter.

597
598
599

600–602. From the list on the left select the statement which describes the action of each structure listed on the right.

A. Connects the muscles to the brain.
B. Connects the eyes to the brain
C. Connects two different neurons
D. Connects the brain to the muscles
E. Connects the skin to the brain

600. Motor pathway
601. Sensory pathway
602. Connector neuron.

600
601
602

603–605. From the list on the left select the part supplied by the nerves listed on the right.

A. Extensors of the wrist	603. Axillary		603
B. Shoulder muscles	604. Median		604
C. Muscles of the hand	605. Radial.		605
D. Thumb			
E. Flexors of the elbow			

10

The special senses

The special senses are sight, hearing, taste, smell, touch, pain and temperature. The tongue, nose and skin have already been discussed. This chapter will deal with the eye and the ear.

THE EYE AND VISION

The eye is the organ of sight. It is concerned with receiving rays of light reflected from the objects in the environment. The nerve endings in the eyeball are stimulated by the light. The optic nerve carries these impulses back to the occipital lobes of the cerebral cortex where they are interpreted.

The eyeball

The eyeballs are almost spherical in shape. They lie in the cone-shaped orbits in the skull, protected by the eyelids in front and by a pad of fat at the back.

Each eyeball is attached to the orbit by six small muscles which move the eyes in all directions. These muscles act together so that both eyeballs move simultaneously in the same direction. If there is a weakness of one muscle, the eye will squint. This is called a *strabismus*.

Dissecting an eyeball is rather like cutting through an onion, only it is not solid the whole way through,. There are only three

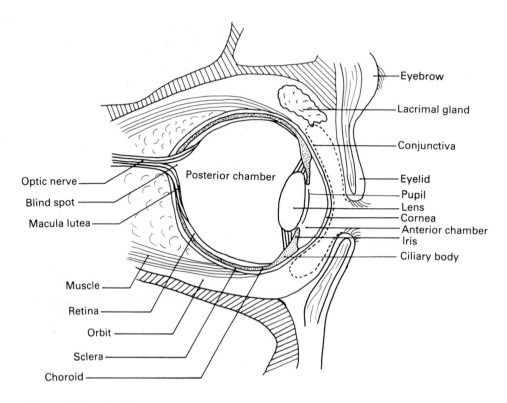

Fig. 10.1 The eyeball in the orbit

coats and the centre is a chamber filled with a jelly-like substance. The coats, from the outer coat inwards, are the *sclera*, the *choroid* and the *retina*.

The sclera and cornea

The outer coat of the eyeball is tough and fibrous and is protective in function. It maintains the shape of the eyeball and provides attachment for the muscles. It consists of two parts. The larger posterior part is opaque. It forms the white part of the eye and is called the *sclera*. The anterior part is transparent. It is the window-like structure called the *cornea*. The cornea allows the rays of light to pass into the eyeball. It is very sensitive and the slightest spot of dust touching it will cause the eyelid to come down like a shutter. This blinking action helps to keep the eyeball clean.

The choroid

The choroid is the coloured part of the eyeball. It is rich in blood vessels and is dark brown in colour. This dark colour prevents the rays of light which have entered the eye from being reflected back out again.

The choroid lines the sclera and forms the *iris*, the coloured part of the eyeball. The iris lies between the cornea and the *lens*. It is like a circular curtain with a hole in the middle called the *pupil*. Behind the iris is a circular muscle called the *ciliary body*. This muscle has ligaments attached to it which hold the lens in place. The ciliary body by contracting and relaxing, can alter the shape of the lens. It secretes a watery fluid called *aqueous humour* which is contained in the *anterior chamber* of the eyeball. The anterior chamber is the space between the cornea and the lens.

The lens is a colourless, transparent, biconvex elastic structure. It lies between the aqueous humour and the vitreous humour which is the jelly-like substance contained in the *posterior chamber* of the eyeball.

The retina

The retina is the nervous coat of the eyeball. It consists of a pigmented layer of tissue which attaches it to the choroid. In front of this tissue is a network of nerve cells and fibres and a layer of light sensitive cells called *rods* and *cones*.

There are millions of rods and cones in each eyeball. Most of the cones are clustered together at the back of the retina where they form a very sensitive area called the *macula lutea*. When you look directly at something, the rays of light from that object are focused on the centre of the macula and the object appears clearer than its surroundings. Look at the wall above a clock. You can see that the clock is there but you will not be able to tell the time until you look directly at it.

The cones are sensitive to bright light and colour. The rods are sensitive to dim light and they contain a substance called *visual purple*. Visual purple prevents night blindness and requires the intake of vitamin A to maintain its effectiveness (see p. 100).

Beside the macula is the *blind spot*. This is where the *optic nerve* leaves the eye and there are no nerve cells. We do not see it as a blind spot because we see with both eyes at once. One eye compensates for the blind spot of the other.

The optic nerve from each eyeball passes back into the skull and they come together at the base of the brain. Some of the nerve fibres cross at this point so that the nerves which eventually reach the right and left occipital cortex contain fibres from both eyes.

Seeing with both eyes (binocular vision) produces three-dimensional vision. Try shutting one eye. Everything looks flat. Now open the other eye and the objects you are looking at will appear to stand out. You can judge distance, height and depth much better. It is called stereoscopic vision.

Vision

When rays of light pass from one substance to another of different density, they bend. If you stand a stick in a pool of water the stick will look as if it bends as it enters the water. This bending of light rays is called refraction and is the reason why we can see. Light rays entering the eyeball pass through the cornea, the aqueous humour, the lens and the vitreous humour. These substances all bend the rays so that they become focused on the retina.

The lens is adjustable allowing the rays of light to be bent as necessary. If you are looking at a close object the rays must be bent through a greater angle than if you are looking at a distant object (see Fig. 10.2). For reading, therefore, the lens must be thicker. The ciliary muscle contracts and the lens becomes more convex. Lifting the head and looking into the distance relaxes the muscle and keeps the eyes from

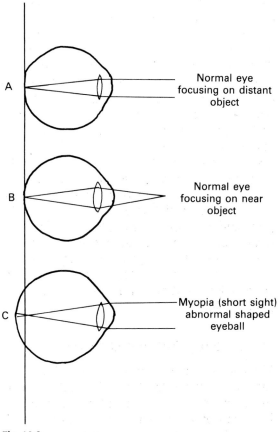

A Normal eye focusing on distant object

B Normal eye focusing on near object

C Myopia (short sight) abnormal shaped eyeball

Fig. 10.2

getting too tired. Sometimes the lens become hardened in the centre and is opaque. A white spot appears on the lens. It is called *cataract* and is a common cause of blindness in old age.

Focusing the eyes is called *accommodation*. Accommodation depends on the shape of the lens, movement of the eyes and the size of the pupil. As one gets older, the ability to focus on close object gets difficult and spectacles must be used for reading. Individuals with long or short sight (*myopia*) require glasses because the eyeball is not quite the right shape.

The muscle fibres of the iris are circular and radiating. When the radiating muscle fibres contract under the influence of the sympathetic nervous system, the pupils dilate and more light enters the eyes. When the circular fibres contract, the pupil constricts and less light enters. The circular muscle fibres are influenced by the parasympathetic nervous system. The iris is like a shutter of a camera, allowing more light to enter when the light is dull and less if the light is bright.

Certain drugs have an effect on the size of the pupil. Morphine constricts it and atropine dilates it. Homatropine drops are occasionally instilled into the eye to allow the doctor to get a better view of the retina with an ophthalmoscope. When nursing patients with head injuries, accurate observations must be made of the size of each pupil as their reactions are of great value in diagnosis. As the damaged brain swells, pressure inside the skull builds up. This pressure displaces and damages the cranial nerve which supplies the pupil and the pupil on the side of the damaged brain dilates. The nurse, observing that the patient with a head injury has unequal pupils, must report her findings immediately as surgical intervention at this stage may save the patient's life.

The structures which protect the eye

The eye is a very delicate organ and it is protected by several structures. The fact that it lies in a bony cavity which is softened at the back by a pad of fat prevents direct injury. In old age and long and serious illnesses, the pads of fat diminish and give the person a hollow-eyed appearance. On the other hand, in exophthalmic goitre the pad of fat enlarges and pushes the eyeball forwards.

The other structures which give protection are the eyelids, the eyebrows and the tear glands

The *eyelids* are like shutters. They are muscular and are covered with skin, and can be opened and closed at will. However, if an object approaches the eye suddenly, the lids automatically close and the eyelashes help to sweep the object away.

Covering the front of the eyeball and lining the eyelids is a thin layer of transparent mucous membrane called the *conjunctiva*. Any insect or speak of dust which has not been swept away by the eyelashes will stick to the conjunctiva and can be removed without damaging the eye itself. Drugs given into the eye as drops or ointments should be placed gently into the lower conjunctival sac.

The *eyebrows* help to cut down the amount of light entering the eye. This is why we frown when the light is too bright. They also prevent sweat from running down into the eyes.

A foreign body in the eye makes you 'weep', not because it is so painful but more as a reflex attempt to wash away the irritating object. Situated above each eye is a small gland called the *lacrymal gland*. This gland secretes tears. Tears are a salty fluid which flows over the front of the eye, continually washing it. Tears contain a substance called *lysozyme* which kills off any micro-organisms. Normally the tears flow towards the nasal side of the eye where they enter the *lacrymal sac* before passing down the *lacrymal duct* and being evaporated in the nose. It is only when the eye is injured or when we are emotionally upset that we are aware of the tears. The lacrymal gland then produces additional fluid which overflows and runs down the cheeks.

THE EAR

The ear is the organ of hearing. It is constructed in such a way that the sound waves

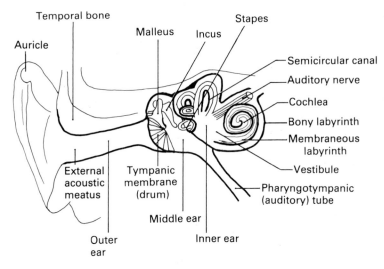

Fig. 10.3 The ear

passing through the atmosphere are caught up and transmitted to the hearing centre in the temporal lobe of the cerebral cortex. The ear also plays a part in maintaining balance. It consists of three parts—the external, middle and internal ear.

The external ear

The visible part of the ear is the *auricle*. The auricle is a collecting trumpet for the sound waves. It is of more use to the lower animals than to man as they can move the auricle towards the source of the sound. The auricle is composed of elastic fibrocartilage covered with skin.

The more important parts of the ear lie within the temporal bone. From the auricle a curved canal, the external *acoustic meatus*, leads towards the ear drum. This canal is partly cartilage and partly bone. It is lined with skin from which hairs grow, and it contains small glands which secrete wax. The curve in the canal, the hairs and the wax are all protective in function and help to prevent foreign bodies from reaching the ear drum.

Over-secretion of wax causes deafness. The wax can be syringed out of the ear. This is a fairly simple procedure, but it must be done by the doctor or by a specialist nurse because

of the danger of perforating the delicate drum. During syringing or inspection of the ear, the canal can be straightened out by pulling the auricle backwards and upwards.

The external acoustic meatus ends at the *tympanic membrane* which is the ear drum. The tympanic membrane is composed of fibrous tissue covered with a modified skin. It separates the external ear from the middle ear.

The middle ear

The middle ear is an irregular space in the temporal bone. It is sometimes called the tympanic cavity. It is lined with mucous membrane and contains air which reaches it through the *pharyngotympanic* or *auditory tube*. The air, at atmospheric pressure, is equal on both sides of the tympanic membrane and allows it to vibrate. Problems arise when the pressures are unequal, as occurs in an aircraft which is not pressurised. The ears will 'pop', hearing will be affected and there may be quite severe pain in the ear as the plane takes off or lands. Chewing and swallowing help to keep the auditory tube open.

The lining of the auditory tube is continuous with the nasopharynx so that middle ear infection, or *otitis media*, can complicate a cold in the nose or a sore throat. If pus collects in the middle ear, its only way of escape is by rupturing the tympanic membrane with serious results.

The tympanic membrane forms the lateral wall of the tympanic cavity. The medial wall separates the middle ear from the internal ear. It is a thin plate of bone in which there are two windows. The *round window* is covered by a membrane which bulges out when the *oval window* moves in. The oval window is occluded by part of one of the auditory ossicles.

The auditory ossicles

Three small bones called the auditory ossicles extend across the middle ear from the tympanic membrane to the oval window. These bones are shaped like a hammer, an anvil and a stirrup and are called *malleus, incus* and *stapes* respectively. The handle of the malleus is in contact with the tympanic membrane and the base of stapes is in contact with the oval window. The incus lies in between and articulates with both the other bones.

The internal ear

The internal ear is a complicated arrangement of passages hollowed out of the temporal bone. It is called the *bony labyrinth* and consists of three parts; the *vestibule*, the *semicircular canals* and the *cochlea*. The three semicircular canals open out of the vestibule which is the part next to the middle ear. The

cochlea also opens out of the vestibule. It is shaped like a snail's shell.

The bony labyrinth is full of fluid in which floats the membraneous labyrinth. The membraneous labyrinth is the same shape as the bony labyrinth but somewhat smaller. It also contains fluid in which are the hairlike endings of the *auditory nerve*. The auditory nerve has two branches. One branch goes to the cochlea, this is the nerve of hearing. The other smaller branch supplies the semicircular canals which are concerned with balance.

HEARING AND BALANCE

Waves of sound pass into the acoustic meatus and hit the tympanic membrane which then vibrates. These vibrations are conveyed through the auditory ossicles to the oval window. The oval window vibrates and sets up waves in the fluid in the cochlea. This moves the fluid in the membraneous labyrinth and the nerve endings are stimulated. The impulses are then transmitted to the temporal lobe of the cerebral cortex where they are appreciated as sound.

The nerve endings in the semicircular canals are stimulated by the pressure of the fluid changing with the different positions of the head in space. They have nothing to do with hearing but they play some part in maintaining balance. Over stimulation of this branch of the auditory nerve will cause giddiness or vertigo.

The special senses questions

Diagrams—Questions 606–626

606–617. The eye

A. Cornea
B. Lacrimal gland
C. Pupil
D. Retina
E. Aqueous humour
F. Vitreous humour
G. Lens
H. Ciliary body
I. Conjunctiva
J. Optic nerve
K. Choroid
L. Iris

606
607
608
609
610
611
612
613
614
615
616
617

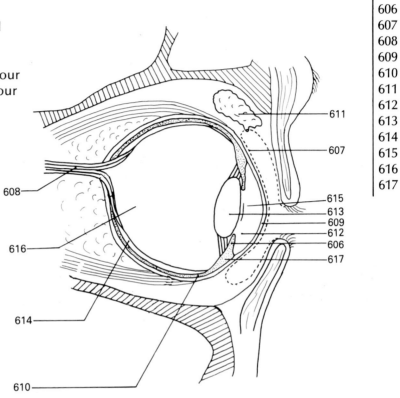

618–626. The ear

A. Auricle
B. External acoustic meatus
C. Tympanic membrane
D. Middle ear
E. Malleus
F. Incus
G. Stapes
H. Cochlea
I. Semicircular canals

618
619
620
621
622
623
624
625
626

Questions 627–630 are of the multiple choice type.

627. **The number of muscles attaching each eye to the orbit is:**
    A. 2
    B. 4
    C. 6
    D. 8.

628. **Which one of the following parts of the eyeball is the white part?**
    A. Cornea
    B. Choroid
    C. Retina
    D. Sclera.

629. **The iris is a part of one of the following parts of the eyeball. Which one?**
    A. Cornea
    B. Choroid
    C. Retina
    D. Sclera.

630. **Which one of the following has no refractive power?**
    A. Aqueous humour
    B. Cornea
    C. Lens
    D. Sclera.

Questions 631–666 are of the true/false type.   T | F |

631–634. The orbit is :
    631. cone-shaped
    632. spherical
    633. part of the eyeball
    634. part of the skull.

635–638. The lens is :
    635. attached to the ciliary body
    636. biconcave
    637. elastic
    638. transparent.

639–642. Accommodation involves the :
    639. movement of the eye
    640. shape of the lens
    641. size of the pupil
    642. the blind spot.

643–646. The conjunctiva :
    643. covers the front of the eyeball
    644. lines the orbit
    645. lines the eyelids
    646. secretes tears.

647–650. The external acoustic meatus :
    647. lies entirely within the temporal bone
    648. is lined with mucous membrane
    649. is a straight tube
    650. ends at the tympanic membrane.

651–654. The middle ear :
    651. is connected to the nasopharynx
    652. contains the semicircular canals
    653. contains air at atmospheric pressure
    654. contains wax-secreting glands.

655–658. The internal ear :
    655. is a cavity in the temporal bone
    656. is the bony labyrinth
    657. contains the auditory ossicles
    658. contains fluid.

659–662. The cochlea :   T | F

    659. consists of three circular canals
    660. contains the endings of the auditory nerve
    661. is concerned with hearing
    662. is concerned with balance.

663–666. We can hear because :

    663. sounds travel in waves
    664. the incus is in contact with the oval window
    665. pressure is exerted on the nerve endings in the semicircular canals
    666. the tympanic membrane vibrates.

Questions 667–681 are of the matching items type.

667–669. From the list on the left select a statement which describes each structure listed on the right.

A. Is composed of voluntary muscle tissue	667. Iris	667
B. Is composed of involuntary muscle tissue	668. Lens	668
C. Is highly elastic	669. Pupil.	669
D. Dilates in dim light		
E. Is attached to the retina		

670–672. From the list on the left select a statement which describes each structure listed on the right.

A. Secretes tears	670. Macula lutea	670
B. Sensitive to dim light	671. Rods	671
C. Part of the choroid	672. Lacrimal gland	672
D. Consists of cones		
E. Gives stereoscopic vision		

673–675. From the list on the left select the abnormality which results in the conditions on the right.

A. A weak eye muscle	673. Myopia	673
B. An abnormal cornea	674. Cataract	674
C. A detached retina	675. Strabismus.	675
D. Hardening of the lens		
E. An abnormal shaped eyeball		

676–678. From the list on the left select the statement which describes each part of the ear listed on the right.

A. Is made of hyaline cartilage	676. External	676
B. Lies only partly in the temporal bone	677. Internal	677
C. Contains the openings into the auditory tube	678. Middle.	678
D. Contains the semicircular canals		
E. Contains mastoid air cells		

679–681. From the list on the left select the statement which describes the structures on the right.

A. Is shaped like a stirrup	679. Incus	679
B. Is the middle auditory ossicle	680. Malleus	680
C. Is floating in lymph	681. Stapes.	681
D. Is in contact with the cochlea		
E. Is in contact with the tympanic membrane		

11

The endocrine system

Have you ever wondered why some of your friends are always doing something in their free time whilst others just go to bed or are content to sit around gossiping? What makes you want to stay at home to watch the television when your friends are all urging you to go out jogging? Why are you too frightened to open your mouth in class whilst Nurse Black is always interrupting the tutor? Why do some people never feel the cold, even in the middle of winter?

What makes us all different? Inheritance, background, upbringing and endocrine glands all play a part in making us what we are.

The endocrine glands are very complex and many of their functions are not yet completely understood. Unlike the sweat and digestive glands, they do not have ducts to carry their secretions to the parts where they are required. The secretions of the endocrine glands go straight into the blood capillaries. This is why they are called ductless glands. Their secretions or *hormones* are called internal secretions.

The following are the glands of the endocrine system:

pituitary
thyroid
parathyroid
adrenal
pancreas
pineal
ovaries and testes.

THE PITUITARY GLAND (HYPOPHYSIS CEREBRI)

The pituitary gland is a small gland about the size and shape of a cherry. It lies in the skull at the base of the brain to which it is attached. It consists of an anterior and a posterior lobe.

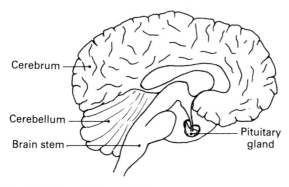

Fig. 11.1 The pituitary gland

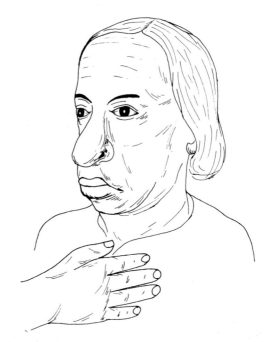

Fig. 11.2 Acromegaly

The anterior lobe

The anterior lobe produces several hormones and has some control over the activities of other glands.

The *growth* hormone affects the growth of all cells, including the cells of the epiphyses of long bones. In childhood, undersecretion of the hormone results in stunted growth and the child becomes a *dwarf*. The nervous system is not affected and the dwarf is not retarded mentally. Recently, these children have been treated with injections of human growth hormone and they have gone on to develop normally. A child with oversecretion of this hormone will grow abnormally tall (*gigantism*). In adults, oversecretion results in thickening of the hands, feet and skull (*acromegaly*).

The other hormones from the anterior lobe of the pituitary gland regulate the actions of the other glands.

The *thyroid stimulating hormone* (T.S.H.) controls the thyroid gland.

The *adrenocorticotrophic hormone* (A.C.T.H.) controls the cortex of the adrenal glands.

The *gonadotrophic hormone* controls the sex glands.

The posterior lobe

The posterior lobe of the pituitary gland produces a secretion known as *pituitrin*. Pituitrin contains two hormones: *oxytocin* and *vasopressin*.

Oxytocin is released at the onset of labour. It contracts the pregnant uterus and under its influence the breasts will produce milk.

Vasopressin has an anti-diuretic effect. It controls the amount of water excreted by the kidneys. It also stimulates involuntary muscles to contract and acts on the walls of the arterioles causing them to constrict and so raises the blood pressure.

THE THYROID GLAND

The thyroid gland consists of two lobes, one on either side of the larynx and joined by a narrow piece of tissue called the isthmus. It is normally invisible but, if enlarged, it can form an obvious swelling at the base of the neck called a *goitre*.

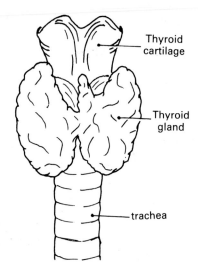

Fig. 11.3   Thyroid gland

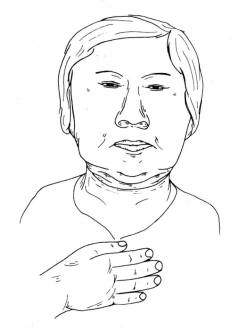

Fig. 11.4   Myxoedema

The thyroid gland consists of numerous follicles held together by connective tissue. It has a very rich blood supply. The follicles contain a yellow jelly-like fluid called the colloid. Iodine is required in the diet for the proper development of the colloid and the hormone *thyroxine*. Thyroxine is developed and stored in the colloid.

Thyroxine has many functions. It controls the rate of metabolism. It is necessary for normal mental and physical development and for healthy hair and skin.

If the thyroid gland is underactive (*hypothyroidism*), the individual will be lethargic and slow in his movements and thoughts. He will be fat and puffy in appearance with coarse dry hair and skin. His basic metabolic rate will be low and he is said to suffer from *myxoedema*. A child with hypothyroidism is called a *cretin*. He is a dwarf with dry skin, straight black hair and a prominent abdomen. He is mentally deficient and has a tongue which is too long for his mouth. Fortunately, both the cretin and the adult with myxoedema can be treated by giving thyroxine by mouth.

An overactive thyroid gland (*hyperthyroidism*) produces an overactive individual. He burns up his fuel foods at a terrific rate, has a good appetite but is always thin. His eyes may protrude (exophthalmus) and he is very

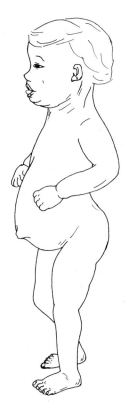

Fig. 11.5   A cretin

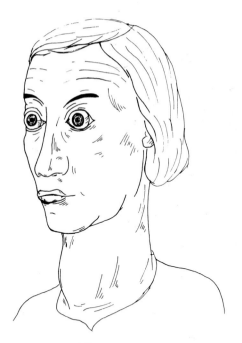

Fig. 11.6 Hyperthyroidism

nervous and excitable. He has a rapid pulse rate and is always warm as he makes so much heat in his body because of his high metabolic rate. There are various treatments for patients with hyperthyroidism. They may be treated with drugs which inhibit the uptake of iodine by the gland, with radio-active iodine which will destroy the cells of the gland and by surgical removal of the gland.

Calcitonin is another hormone from the thyroid gland. Its function is to maintain the correct amount of calcium in the blood.

THE PARATHYROID GLANDS

There are four little parathyroid glands situated at the back of the thyroid gland. The hormone they produce (*parathormone*) acts with calcitonin to maintain the correct amount of calcium in the blood and in the bones.

If these glands are overactive, the amount of calcium in the bones is reduced and they become soft, painful and easily fractured. Under-secretion of the hormone causes muscular spasm in the hands and feet called tetany.

THE ADRENAL OR SUPRARENAL GLANDS

There are two adrenal glands, one situated above each kidney. These glands consist of two parts, a cortex on the outside and a medulla in the centre.

The adrenal cortex

A number of different hormones are secreted by the adrenal cortex. They are called *corticosteroids, cortisol* or simply *steroids*. The function of the steroids is to regulate carbohydrate metabolism. In times of stress, the steroids convert protein and fat into glucose. The steroids are anti-allergic and anti-inflammatory. Synthetic steroids have been developed to treat allergic and inflammatory conditions.

The adrenal cortex also produces a hormone which controls the reabsorption of sodium and water in the kidneys and the excretion of potassium. Over-secretion of this hormone may lead to oedema and high blood pressure. Under-secretion is called *Addison's disease*. In this condition the patient has a low blood pressure, there is loss of sodium and water from the body and he develops muscle weakness, nausea and vomiting. Addison's disease used to be fatal but it can now be treated with steroids.

The other hormones from the adrenal cortex are the sex hormones—*testosterone, oestrogen* and *progesterone*. Over-secretion of these hormones produce sexual changes depending on the age and sex of the individual. A woman may become masculine and a man feminine. A child will reach puberty at a very early age.

The adrenal medulla

The medulla of the adrenal gland produces *adrenalin* and *noradrenalin*. These hormones work in conjunction with the sympathetic nervous system.

The output of adrenalin is increased in times of anxiety and stress, such as prior to an examination or an important interview. The blood pressure shoots up, the pulse is rapid, more oxygen is taken into the lungs and extra glucose is liberated from the store in the liver. The last thing you want is a big meal and you may even feel sick. There is no need to describe the symptoms as everyone is familiar with them. It is comforting to think that this is nature's way of helping us to face up to difficult situations.

THE OVARIES

The ovaries are the female sex glands and will be described in the next chapter. They secrete the hormones which bring about the physiological changes which occur in a girl at puberty, and they maintain the normal menstrual cycle in a woman during her child-bearing years.

THE TESTES

The testes are the male sex glands. The hormone is responsible for the changes occurring in a boy at puberty and for maintaining the normal sex urge in the adult male.

THE PANCREAS

The *islets* of *Langerhans* in the pancreas are endocrine glands. The hormone *insulin* goes straight into the blood stream. Insulin allows the body to store glucose as glycogen. If it is absent or deficient, the patient suffers from diabetes mellitus. In diabetes, glucose cannot be stored, the blood contains too much and it is excreted in the urine.

THE PINEAL GLAND

This is a small gland situated in the brain. Its functions are not yet completely understood but it seems to stimulate the cells in the skin which produce the black pigment called *melanin*.

Endocrine system questions

Questions 682–685 are of the multiple choice type.

682. **Which one of the following is a feature of hypothyroidism?**

    A. Nervous tension
    B. Underweight
    C. Exophthalmus
    D. Lethargy.

683. **Which one of the following is a feature of hyperthyroidism?**

    A. Bradycardia
    B. Raised metabolic rate
    C. Loss of appetite
    D. Coarse hair.

684. **Which one of the following is a feature of undersecretion of the parathyroid gland?**

    A. Soft bones
    B. Fractures
    C. Tetany
    D. Increased metabolic rate.

685. **Which one of the following is a feature of oversecretion of the pituitary gland in an adult?**

    A. Pigmented skin
    B. Large hands
    C. Gigantism
    D. Mental retardation.

Questions 686–717 are of the true/false type.

686–689. Hormones are :

686. similar to enzymes
687. present in blood plasma
688. secreted by glands with ducts
689. substances which stimulate activity in organs.

690–693. The pituitary gland :

690. is attached to the brain
691. has four lobes
692. controls growth
693. controls the other glands.

694–697. Vasopressin :

694. is a hormone from the posterior lobe of the pituitary gland
695. has a diuretic effect
696. raises the blood pressure
697. influences the breast to produce milk.

698–701. Thyroxine :

698. requires iodine for its development
699. is stored in a colloid
700. controls metabolism
701. influences mental development.

702–705. The adrenal cortex :

702. is in the centre of the gland
703. produces adrenalin
704. regulates carbohydrate metabolism
705. is essential for life.

706–709. The parathyroid glands :

706. are four in number
707. secrete calcitonin
708. control the calcium content of the blood
709. produce melanin.

710–713. The reaction of the body to stress involves :

    710. insulin

    711. cortisol

    712. adrenalin

    713. parathormone.

714–717. Adrenalin :

    714. is a steroid

    715. is essential for life

    716. acts in conjunction with the sympathetic nervous system

    717. controls fluid balance.

T   F

Questions 718–723 are of the matching items type.

718–720. From the list on the left select a symptom or sign applicable to each condition listed on the right.

A. A large jaw
B. Muscle weakness
C. A rapid pulse
D. A large tongue
E. Brittle bones

718. A cretin
719. Addison's disease
720. Acromegaly.

718
719
720

721–723. From the list on the left select the condition which produces each disease listed on the right.

A. Overactive parathyroid glands
B. An underactive thyroid glands
C. An enlarged thyroid
D. An underactive pineal gland
E. An underactive pancreas

721. Diabetis mellitus
722. Goitre
723. Myxoedema.

721
722
723

12

The reproductive system

One of the characteristics of life is the ability to reproduce. This can be a simple or a complicated process. One-celled organisms simply divide into two. The parent cell grows and matures until the time comes for it to divide. The two resulting daughter cells are exact replicas of the parent. In this way, the species is continued from generation to generation. Occasionally, spontaneous changes occur in the daughter cells. These are called *mutations*. Sometimes these new cells are an improvement on the parent and they strengthen the species. On the other hand, the reverse may happen and the organism may not survive.

In the higher, multicellular forms of life there is some type of sexual reproduction. Each new creature has two parents, male and female. The essential feature of this method of reproduction is that the female produces the egg cells or ova and the male produces the germ cells or spermatozoa. These two cells must unite to form a completely different individual who inherits some characteristics from both parents (see Ch. 1).

The fertilisation of the human *ovum* by the *spermatozoon* occurs in the mother's body. The resulting *zygote* embeds itself in the wall of the uterus and becomes an *embryo*. The cells of the embryo develop and multiply until in about 8 weeks it has assumed the shape of the human being. By 12 weeks the embryo is referred to as a *fetus*. The fetus remains in the mother's uterus for a further 32 weeks. During this time it grows and develops until it is ca-

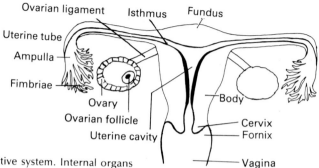

Fig. 12.1 Female reproductive system. Internal organs

pable of a separate existence. The 40 weeks during which the baby is developing in the uterus is called the *gestation period*.

THE FEMALE REPRODUCTIVE SYSTEM

In the female the reproductive organs are in two groups—internal and external. The internal organs consist of the ovaries, the uterus and the vagina.

The external organs are collectively called the vulva.

The internal organs

The ovaries

The ovaries are the female gonads or sex glands. They produce the ova and also the sex hormones. They do not begin to function until the girl reaches puberty at the age of 12 to 14 years.

The ovaries are small almond-shaped glands, about 2 to 3 cm long. They are situated in the pelvic cavity, one on either side of the uterus. They consist of two layers, the outer cortex and the inner medulla which is composed of fibrous tissue.

The *cortex* of the ovary consists of germinal epithelium which contains the ovarian *follicles*. Each ovarian follicle contains fluid and an immature ovum. At puberty and every 28 days from then until the menopause (about 50 years of age) one follicle comes to the surface, bursts and expels its ovum which is now mature. The ovum finds its way into the uterus where it may or may not be fertilised. After the

follicle has ruptured, it becomes the *corpus luteum* which remains throughout pregnancy. If pregnancy does not occur, the corpus luteum degenerates and becomes a fibrous scar on the surface of the ovary.

The ovum produces the female sex hormones—oestrogen and progesterone. These are responsible for the physical and mental changes in the adolescent girl and also for the preparation of the uterus and breasts for pregnancy. *Oestrogen* comes from the *ovarian follicle* and *progesterone* from the *corpus luteum*.

The uterus

The uterus is a hollow organ about 10 cm long. It is situated in the pelvic cavity between the rectum and the bladder. Projecting from it on either side are two tubes called the uterine tubes.

The uterus has a thick muscular coat which thins out as it expands in pregnancy. The non-pregnant uterus is pear-shaped. The broad upper part lying between the uterine tubes is the *fundus*. The main part is called the *body*. This narrows inferiorly to form the *cervix* or neck which projects down into the vagina. The opening from the body into the cervix is the internal *os* and the opening into the vagina is the external *os*.

The uterus and uterine tubes are covered by a fold of the peritoneum called the broad ligament. This part of the peritoneum is reflected from the upper surface of the urinary bladder, over the uterus and up over the rectum. It helps to hold the uterus in place. The broad

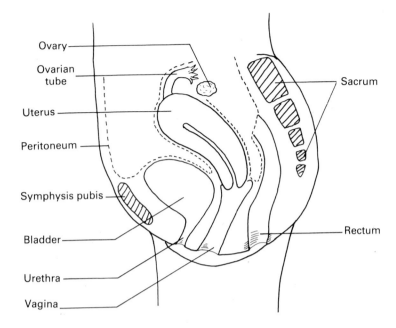

Ovary
Ovarian tube
Uterus
Peritoneum
Symphysis pubis
Bladder
Urethra
Vagina
Sacrum
Rectum

Fig. 12.2   The pelvic organs

ligament and the round ligament, which extends from the uterus to the vulva, hold the uterus in a position of antiversion and antiflexion. This means that it leans forwards and is bent almost at right angles over the bladder.

The uterus is lined with a mucous membrane called the *endometrium*. The blood supply is from the uterine artery, a branch of the iliac artery. Its nerve supply is from the autonomic nervous system.

The uterine tubes are muscular and are lined with ciliated epithelium. They are narrow where they leave the uterus. This part is called the *isthmus* and the wider part is the *ampulla*. The ends of the tubes have fringe-like projections called *fimbriae*. These pass through the posterior fold of the broad ligament into the peritoneal cavity and one long fimbria lies near the corresponding ovary. The uterus is outside the peritoneal cavity but the ovaries lie inside.

Peritonitis or inflammation of the peritoneal cavity is more common in women than in men because of this opening into the peritoneal cavity. Infection can spread upwards from the vagina and uterus into the uterine tubes. *Salpingitis* is inflammation of the uterine tubes.

Fertilisation usually occurs in the ampulla. The zygote is moved along by the cilia into the uterus. Sometimes it stays in the tube and develops there. This is called an *ectopic pregnancy*.

The vagina

The vagina is the passage leading from the uterus to the external organs. It is a flattened, muscular tube lined with stratified squamous epithelium. Where the cervix enters the vagina are the *fornices*. The anterior, posterior and two lateral fornices form a continuous circular recess between the cervix and the vagina. The exit of the vagina is in the vulva behind the urethral orifice. The hymen is the membrane which partially occludes the vaginal orifice. It has no known function.

The vulva or external genitalia

The term vulva covers all parts of the external genitals. The *labia majora* are two thick folds of skin and fat on which coarse hair grows at

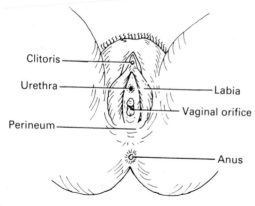

Fig. 12.3 External genitals

the onset of puberty. Lying between them are the *labia minora*, two smaller folds of skin containing many sebaceous glands. Where these folds meet anteriorly is the *clitoris* which corresponds to the penis in the male. The clitoris is a very sensitive organ.

The *vestibule* between the labia minora is where the vaginal and urethral orifices are situated. The *vestibular glands* secrete mucus which lubricates the vagina.

It is frequently quite difficult to catheterise a female patient, especially if she has had children and the vaginal orifice has been stretched or torn. The urethral orifice can be difficult to find. Great care must be taken when swabbing

the vulva and inserting the catheter to ensure the sterility of the procedure.

THE MENSTRUAL CYCLE

From puberty to the menopause a series of changes occur in the uterus, usually every 28 days. This is called the menstrual cycle. It is controlled by the ovarian hormones which in turn are stimulated by the gonadotrophic hormones from the anterior lobe of the pituitary gland.

The menstrual period, which is the shedding of the endometrium by the uterus, lasts for about 5 days. For the next 9 days the hormone oestrogen repairs the lining and causes the endometrium to thicken. On the fourteenth day *ovulation* takes place. A follicle bursts and liberates a mature ovum. The follicle now becomes the corpus luteum which secretes progesterone. Progesterone causes the endometrium to thicken and a watery mucus is produced. This is preparing the uterus to receive a fertilised ovum (see Fig. 12.4).

If fertilisation takes place, progesterone continues to be secreted and the menstrual cycle stops for the 40 weeks of pregnancy. If fertilisation does not occur, the corpus luteum ceases to function and the endometrium is

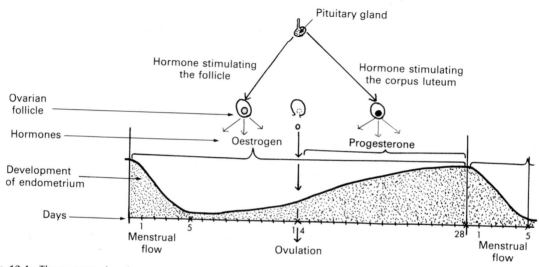

Fig. 12.4 The menstrual cycle

shed. This debris passes out of the uterus via the vagina in the form of a discharge of blood and dead cells. The first day of the next cycle has begun.

THE MAMMARY GLANDS

The mammary glands or breasts are accessory glands of the female reproductive system. They are present in both sexes but only develop in the female.

The breasts develop at puberty when they are influenced by the ovarian hormones. They only function after the birth of a child when they are stimulated to produce milk by the hormones from the pituitary gland.

Each gland consists of a number of lobes with ducts which reach the surface at the nipple. These ducts are called the lactiferous ducts. They are supported by fibrous tissue and fat. The amount of adipose tissue determines the size of the breasts.

THE MALE REPRODUCTIVE SYSTEM

The male reproductive system is responsible for the production of the spermatozoon or male germ cell and for projecting it into the female vagina. The spermatozoa are small cells with long tails. The tail gives the cell mobility and drives it up through the uterus into the uterine tubes where it may fuse with an ovum. Enormous numbers of these cells are liberated at one time.

The male genital organs are the testes, the deferent and ejaculatory ducts, the penis, the seminal vesicles and the prostate gland.

The testes

The testes are the glands which produce the *spermatozoa* and the male sex hormone *testosterone*. Testosterone produces the characteristic changes in a boy at puberty. The secretion of testosterone is stimulated by the gonadotrophic hormone from the anterior lobe of the pituitary gland.

Puberty occurs later in a boy than a girl. The boy is between 13 to 16 years old before his voice breaks, hair grows on his face and body and the genital organs enlarge. At this time, the testes are activated to produce spermatozoa.

The two testes lie outside the body in the *scrotum*. The scrotum is a sac of thin dark-coloured skin lying behind the penis.

The testes develop in the fetus on the posterior wall of the abdomen and they descend into the scrotum before birth. They descend through the inguinal canal in the groin carrying with them part of the peritoneum which remains as a covering. They also carry with them the ducts, the blood vessels and the nerves. These structures form the spermatic cords which suspend the testes in the scrotum.

The spermatozoa develop most successfully at a temperature below body heat. This is achieved by the testes being outside the body.

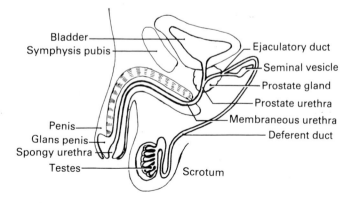

Fig. 12.5 Male reproductive organs

A testis which has failed to descend is one of the causes of infertility in a man.

Each testis consists of two or three hundred lobules. Each lobule contains several convoluted tubules in which the spermatozoa are produced. From the tubules the germ cells pass through a series of twisted ducts into the *deferent duct* which carries the spermatozoa up through the spermatic cord into the pelvis. Between the tubules are the interstitial cells which secrete *testosterone*.

The seminal vesicles

The seminal vesicles are two small sacs which lie at the back of the bladder. The lining of these structures secretes a fluid called *seminal fluid* which helps to nourish the spermatozoa. Each seminal vesicle has a short duct which joins up with the corresponding deferent duct to form the *ejaculatory ducts*. The ejaculatory ducts pass through the prostate gland and join the urethra.

The prostate gland

The prostate gland produces a thin lubricating fluid. It lies at the base of the bladder and surrounds the urethra. This gland may become enlarged in old age when it will obstruct the urethra causing acute retention of urine.

The penis

The penis, like the testes, is an external organ. It is the common passage for semen and urine. The semen is a fluid containing spermatozoa and secretions from the seminal vesicles and the prostate gland.

The urethra is about 20 cm long. It is called the prostate urethra where it leaves the bladder and passes through the prostate gland. It then becomes the membraneous urethra in the perineal region. The third part lies in the penis and is called the spongy urethra. There are two urethral sphincter muscles. The internal sphincter lies at the neck of the bladder and the external sphincter is in the membraneous part of the urethra.

The penis consists of three columns of erectile tissue and involuntary muscle tissue covered with skin. It has a rich blood supply and when engorged with blood it becomes enlarged and erect. The tip of the penis is a bulbous structure called the *glans penis*. This is partially covered by a fold of skin called the *prepuce*. The prepuce or foreskin should be loose. If tight it may have to be cut. The operation is called a circumcision. It is done to prevent infection but also for religious reasons.

Reproductive system questions

Diagrams—Questions 724–753

724–730. The female reproductive system

   A. Uterus
   B. Vagina
   C. Ovary
   D. Uterine tube
   E. Urethra
   F. Rectum
   G. Symphysis pubis

724
725
726
727
728
729
730

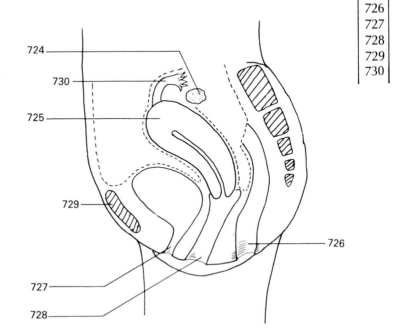

731–736. The external female genitalia

   A. Anus
   B. Clitoris
   C. Labia
   D. Perineum
   E. Vaginal orifice
   F. Urethral orifice

731
732
733
734
735
736

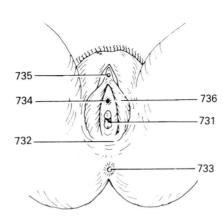

737–746. The uterus and ovaries

A. Fundus
B. Body
C. Fornix
D. External os
E. Cervix
F. Endometrium
G. Fimbriae
H. Ampulla
I. Mature ovarian follicle
J. Germinal epithelium

737
738
739
740
741
742
743
744
745
746

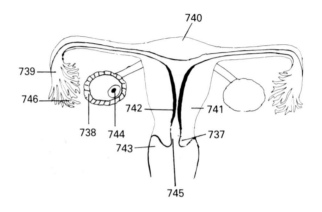

747–753. Male reproductive organs

A. Prostate gland
B. Seminal vesicles
C. Scrotum
D. Testes
E. Deferent duct
F. Symphysis pubis
G. Glans penis

747
748
749
750
751
752
753

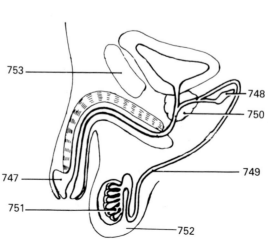

Questions 754–760 are of the multiple choice type.

754. **The vulva consists of all but one of the following parts. Which one?**

    A. Clitoris
    B. Labia minora
    C. Perineum
    D. Vestibule.

755. **Which one of the following is a characteristic of the corpus luteum? It :**

    A. contains the mature ovum
    B. secretes progesterone
    C. is not influenced by the pituitary gland
    D. becomes the ovarian follicle.

756. **Which one of the following cells has only 23 chromosomes?**

    A. A fertilised ovum
    B. An ordinary body cell
    C. A gamete
    D. Any of the cells of the embryo.

757. **On which one of the following days of the menstrual cycle does ovulation occur?**

    A. 5th
    B. 10th
    C. 14th
    D. 28th.

758. **About which week of gestation does the embryo become a fetus?**

    A. 4
    B. 12
    C. 16
    D. 32.

759. **Which one of the following is a function of the deferent duct? It :**

    A. carries semen to the penis
    B. carries spermatozoa to the seminal vesicles
    C. carries testosterone to the blood stream
    D. is a common passage for urine and semen.

760. **The interstitial cells of the testes secrete one of the following :**

    A. gonadotrophic hormone
    B. semen
    C. spermatozoa
    D. testosterone.

Questions 761–788 are of the true/false type.

761–764. The uterus :

    761. lies inside the peritoneal cavity
    762. is covered by the peritoneum
    763. is supported by the bladder
    764. lies in a position of anteversion.

765–768. The uterine tubes :

    765. are broadest where they leave the uterus
    766. are lined with ciliated mucous membrane
    767. penetrate the peritoneum
    768. move the ovum by muscle contraction.

769–772. The ovaries :

    769. are pelvic organs
    770. lie inside the peritoneal cavity
    771. are attached to the uterus by the round ligament
    772. are about 5 cm long.

773–776. The ovarian follicles :

    773. contain the ova
    774. secrete oestrogen
    775. secrete progesterone
    776. become the corpus luteum.

777–780. The testes :

    777. are covered by part of the peritoneum
    778. develop in the abdomen
    779. consist of two lobules
    780. are contained in the scrotum.

781–784. Semen contains :

    781. spermatozoa
    782. seminal fluid
    783. testosterone
    784. prostatic fluid.

785–788. The spermatic cord consists of :

    785. blood vessels
    786. nerves
    787. deferent duct
    788. ejaculatory duct.

Answers

CHAPTER 1 — CELLS, TISSUES and SYSTEMS

Diagrams

1—C	6—E	11—B	16—D
2—B	7—G	12—D	17—F
3—E	8—H	13—I	18—B
4—A	9—A	14—F	19—E
5—D	10—C	15—A	20—C

Multiple choice

21—B	25—B	29—D	33—B
22—B	26—C	30—C	34—A
23—B	27—B	31—C	35—B
24—D	28—C	32—C	

CHAPTER 2 — THE SKELETAL SYSTEM

Diagrams

36—C	49—C	62—C	75—D
37—E	50—D	63—E	76—A
38—A	51—A	64—D	77—D
39—B	52—G	65—A	78—E
40—D	53—F	66—B	79—C
41—D	54—C	67—C	80—B
42—A	55—E	68—B	81—E
43—C	56—B	69—A	82—F
44—B	57—D	70—D	83—A
45—F	58—D	71—E	84—C
46—A	59—A	72—B	85—B
47—E	60—C	73—C	86—D
48—B	61—B	74—A	

Multiple choice

87—C	90—C	92—D	94—B
88—B	91—D	93—A	95—A
89—B			

True/false

96—T	100—F	104—F	108—F
97—F	101—T	105—T	109—F
98—F	102—F	106—T	110—T
99—T	103—T	107—F	111—T

Matching items

112—D	115—A	117—D	119—A
113—C	116—B	118—D	120—E
114—E			

CHAPTER 3 — THE JOINTS and the MUSCLES

Diagrams

121—B	126—C	130—E	134—F
122—C	127—D	131—D	135—C
123—A	128—B	132—A	136—G
124—D	129—H	133—B	137—I
125—A			

Multiple choice

138—C	140—A	142—C	144—D
139—C	141—B	143—C	145—C

True/false

146—T	151—T	156—F	161—T
147—F	152—F	157—T	162—F
148—T	153—T	158—T	163—T
149—F	154—T	159—F	164—F
150—T	155—F	160—T	165—T

Matching items

166—C	169—E	171—B	173—C
167—B	170—A	172—E	174—B
168—D			

CHAPTER 4 — THE CIRCULATORY SYSTEM

Diagrams

175—E	181—D	186—E	191—E
176—B	182—G	187—C	192—G
177—G	183—A	188—F	193—F
178—F	184—B	189—B	194—D
179—A	185—D	190—C	195—A
180—C			

Multiple choice

196—B	199—C	202—C	204—D
197—B	200—A	203—B	205—C
198—B	201—C		

True/false

206—T	218—F	230—T	242—F
207—F	219—T	231—T	243—T
208—T	220—T	232—F	244—T
209—F	221—F	233—F	245—T
210—F	222—F	234—T	246—F
211—F	223—T	235—T	247—T
212—T	224—T	236—F	248—F
213—T	225—T	237—T	249—T
214—T	226—T	238—T	250—T
215—T	227—F	239—T	251—F
216—T	228—T	240—T	252—F
217—F	229—F	241—F	253—F

Matching Items

254—D	257—C	260—E	263—D
255—B	258—D	261—C	264—A
256—C	259—E	262—A	265—E

CHAPTER 5 — THE RESPIRATORY SYSTEM

Diagrams

266—B	270—F	273—D	276—C
267—D	271—A	274—A	277—B
268—G	272—C	275—E	278—F
269—E			

Multiple Choice

279—B	282—C	285—B	287—D
280—B	283—D	286—C	288—B
281—D	284—B		

True/false

289—F	297—T	305—F	313—T
290—T	298—F	306—F	314—F
291—F	299—F	307—F	315—F
292—T	300—T	308—T	316—F
293—T	301—F	309—F	317—T
294—F	302—T	310—T	318—F
295—T	303—F	311—T	319—T
296—F	304—T	312—F	320—T

Matching items

321—E	323—D	325—B	326—D
322—B	324—C		

CHAPTER 6 — THE DIGESTIVE SYSTEM

Diagrams

327—F	334—E	340—B	346—F
328—G	335—G	341—A	347—B
329—A	336—C	342—C	348—C
330—D	337—D	343—E	349—E
331—B	338—A	344—B	350—A
332—C	339—F	345—D	351—D
333—E			

Multiple choice

352—C	355—B	358—B	360—D
353—C	356—D	359—B	361—A
354—D	357—B		

True/false

362—T	372—T	382—F	392—T
363—F	373—T	383—T	393—F
364—T	374—F	384—F	394—F
365—T	375—T	385—T	395—T
366—T	376—F	386—F	396—F
367—F	377—F	387—T	397—T
368—T	378—F	388—F	398—F
369—T	379—T	389—F	399—F
370—F	380—T	390—F	400—T
371—T	381—T	391—T	401—F

Matching items

402—E	406—C	410—E	414—B
403—C	407—E	411—D	415—A
404—D	408—B	412—A	416—D
405—B	409—D	413—B	

CHAPTER 7 — THE SKIN

Diagrams

417—F	419—A	421—C	422—D
418—E	420—B		

Multiple choice

423—B	425—B	427—A	429—C
424—D	426—C	428—A	

True/false

430—F	439—T	448—T	457—F
431—T	440—F	449—F	458—F
432—F	441—T	450—T	459—T
433—T	442—F	451—F	460—T
434—T	443—T	452—T	461—F
435—T	444—F	453—T	462—F
436—T	445—T	454—T	463—T
437—F	446—T	455—F	464—T
438—T	447—T	456—T	465—F

CHAPTER 8 — THE URINARY SYSTEM

Diagrams

466—B	471—D	476—A	480—C
467—A	472—D	477—B	481—B
468—F	473—E	478—F	482—D
469—C	474—C	479—A	483—E
470—E	475—F		

Multiple choice

484—C	486—A	488—B	490—B
485—B	487—C	489—D	491—A

True/false

492—T	496—F	500—F	504—T
493—T	497—T	501—F	505—F
494—F	498—F	502—T	506—T
495—F	499—T	503—T	507—F

Matching items

508—C	509—E	510—A

CHAPTER 9 — THE NERVOUS SYSTEM

Diagrams

511—B	521—K	531—D	541—B
512—D	522—A	532—C	542—E
513—A	523—C	533—F	543—C
514—C	524—E	534—H	544—A
515—B	525—J	535—E	545—D
516—D	526—L	536—C	546—B
517—F	527—A	537—D	547—B
518—H	528—I	538—G	548—D
519—G	529—G	539—F	549—C
520—I	530—B	540—A	550—A

Multiple choice

551—C	553—B	554—C	555—C
552—C			

True/false

556—F	564—T	572—F	580—T
557—T	565—F	573—T	581—F
558—F	566—F	574—F	582—F
559—F	567—T	575—F	583—T
560—T	568—T	576—F	584—F
561—F	569—F	577—T	585—T
562—F	570—T	578—T	586—F
563—T	571—F	579—F	587—T

Matching items

588—C	593—C	598—D	602—C
589—D	594—B	599—C	603—B
590—B	595—D	600—D	604—D
591—E	596—A	601—E	605—A
592—A	597—B		

CHAPTER 10 — THE SPECIAL SENSES

Diagrams

606—L	612—E	617—H	622—H
607—I	613—G	618—A	623—C
608—J	614—D	619—I	624—E
609—A	615—C	620—G	625—F
610—K	616—F	621—D	626—B
611—B			

Multiple choice

627—C	628—D	629—B	630—D

True/false

631—T	640—T	649—F	658—T
632—F	641—T	650—T	659—F
633—F	642—F	651—T	660—T
634—T	643—T	652—F	661—T
635—T	644—F	653—T	662—F
636—F	645—T	654—F	663—T
637—T	646—F	655—T	664—F
638—T	647—F	656—T	665—F
639—T	648—F	657—F	666—T

Matching items

667—B	671—B	675—A	679—B
668—C	672—A	676—B	680—E
669—D	673—E	677—D	681—A
670—D	674—D	678—C	

CHAPTER 11 — THE ENDOCRINE SYSTEM

Multiple choice

682—D		
683—B	684—C	685—B

True/false

686—F	694—T	702—F	710—F
687—T	695—F	703—F	711—T
688—F	696—T	704—T	712—T
689—T	697—F	705—T	713—F
690—T	698—T	706—T	714—F
691—F	699—T	707—F	715—F
692—T	700—T	708—T	716—T
693—T	701—T	709—F	717—F

Matching items

718—D	720—A	722—C	723—B
719—B	721—E		

CHAPTER 12 — THE REPRODUCTIVE SYSTEM

Diagrams

724—C	732—D	740—A	747—G
725—A	733—A	741—B	748—B
726—F	734—F	742—F	749—E
727—E	735—B	743—C	750—A
728—B	736—C	744—I	751—D
729—G	737—E	745—D	752—C
730—D	738—J	746—G	753—F
731—E	739—H		

Multiple choice

754—C	756—C	758—B	760—D
755—B	757—C	759—B	

True/false

761—F	768—F	775—F	782—T
762—T	769—T	776—T	783—F
763—T	770—T	777—T	784—T
764—T	771—F	778—T	785—T
765—F	772—T	779—F	786—T
766—T	773—T	780—T	787—T
767—T	774—T	781—T	788—F

Index